The Nursery Food Book

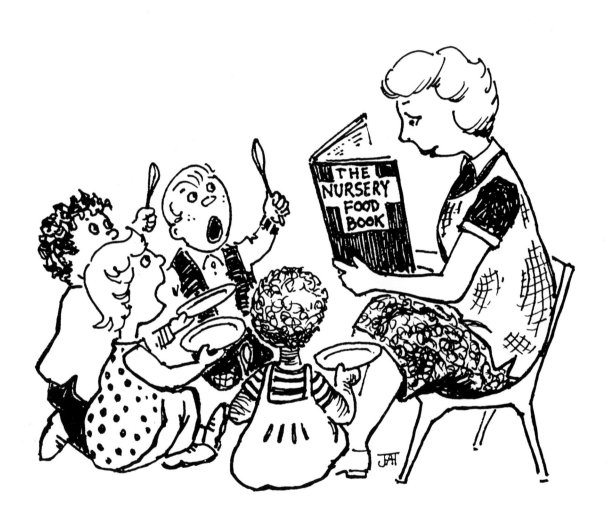

The Nursery Food Book

Mary Whiting and Tim Lobstein

The Food Commission

Cartoons by JAT

Edward Arnold
A member of the Hodder Headline Group
LONDON MELBOURNE AUCKLAND

Edward Arnold is a division of Hodder Headline PLC
338 Euston Road, London NW1 3BH

First published in the United Kingdom 1992

3 5 7 6 4
94 96 98 97 95

British Library Cataloguing in Publication Data
Whiting, Mary
Nursery Food Book
I. Title II. Lobstein, Tim
613.2

ISBN 0-340-55935-7

Typeset in Baskerville by Saxon Printing Ltd, Derby
Printed and bound in the United Kingdom by
The Bath Press, Avon

Preface

This book is about food in nurseries and nursery classes. It aims to answer such questions as:

- What would be a healthy main meal for three year olds?
- What if we have a group of children from mixed cultures?
- What if children only want to eat chips?
- What food activities can young children do?
- What if it's someone's birthday?
- Do we really have to eat coleslaw?

and so on.

This book offers tips, recipes, advice and expertise. It is an invaluable sourcebook for students and handbook for staff.

Acknowledgements

The authors would like to thank:

Helen Strange for her enormous enthusiasm and creative inspiration, and then for reading and enriching our early drafts;

Kathy Adams, Pat Crocker, Barbara Crosby, Sue James and Caroline Skelton for reading and further enriching our drafts;

Esther Mqadi for her generous professional advice and for three delicious Ghanaian recipes;

Chris Carabine for his excellent professional advice;

Sara E. Hill for allowing us to raid her excellent book *More Than Rice And Peas;*

Grub Street Publishers for kindly allowing us to use two mouth-watering recipes from Rosamund Grant's *Caribbean and African Cookery;*

John Whiting for his constant encouragement and willingness to sample any recipe.

We owe a huge debt of gratitude to the many other people working in nursery education who have offered advice, tips, recipes and encouragement.

Contents

— Chapter one —

Every day nutrition
Dangers to health in the modern diet - importance of diet in the early years - dietary guidelines for children under a year old - dietary guidelines for children 1-5 years old - additives.

— Chapter two —

Changing for the better
Summing up what has gone wrong - what can nursery staff do about it? - how to go about making changes: eight tips.

— Chapter three —

What's for dinner?
Sample menus: good and bad - value of snacks - healthy snacks - some psychological considerations - how one nursery started to change - informing parents, and their reactions.

— Chapter four —

Children with eating problems
Children who don't want to eat - children with special diets - children with chewing and swallowing difficulties.

— Chapter five —

A few practicalities
Food hygiene and food poisoning - the safe cooking of meat, poultry and eggs - personal hygiene - ordering food - use of the fridge, the freezer, the microwave - leftovers - the responsibility for hygiene.

— Chapter six —

Multicultural provision
The importance and benefits of this - the value of traditional foods - the responsibility of nurseries and how they can help - food travels around - changing to a multicultural food policy - involving parents - dietary customs - using a taste table - parties and celebrations - feasts and festivals around the year.

— Chapter seven —

Food is fun!
Food pictures - potato printing - playdough - finger painting - papier maché - the home corner - the nursery shop - the nursery café - more special interest tables - games involving food.

— Chapter eight —

Children as cooks
Home-made yogurt, butter, cheese, breads - the child who doesn't want to taste - showing that fish have bones - Scottish herring - suggested sandwich fillings - tossing salads - the question of sharp knives - making soup as a combined activity - ideas for individual cooking: Swedish oat biscuits, fruit yogurt - better cakes - dishing up.

— Chapter nine —

Children as gardeners
The value of growing things - gardening indoors - gardening outdoors - small asphalted play areas - sunless areas - starting from scratch - uses and value of vegetables, fruit, salad crops, herbs and flowers.

— Chapter ten —

Food and basic skills
Language development - mathematical concepts - estimates - time - weighing - measuring - sorting - symmetry - one-to-one correspondence - nursery science - absorbancy, solubility, evaporation - oil and water - oxidation - freezing and melting - plants and daylight - plants and water - oil in nuts - gravity - suspension - music - dance and drama - songs, verses and stories involving food.

— Chapter eleven —

Parties, picnics and outings
Parties - importance of serving good food - the birthday cake - impromptu parties - savoury finger food, spreads and dips - sandwich ideas - sweet dishes - drinks - presentation of party food - picnic food tips - ideas for outings.

RECIPES
THE SLING-IN-THE-BIN LIST
BUDGETING
GETTING HELP
FURTHER READING
USEFUL ADDRESSES
STUDENT ASSIGNMENTS
INDEX

CHAPTER ONE

Everyday Nutrition

———

This chapter is about the principles of healthy eating. It asks:

- What are the problems?
- What can we do about them?
- How should we feed children of different ages?

— Should we be worried? —

By the time we are adults most of us will suffer some form of disease due to our diet. We only have to look in our mouth to see the fillings. A trivial disease, perhaps, but dental services cost the National Health Service (NHS) over £450 million every year.

If we could look at our hearts and arteries and see their condition we might be more alarmed. Heart disease kills a quarter of us, and what we eat contributes greatly to these deaths. Worse still, the age at which heart disease occurs is decreasing – people in their thirties and forties are having heart attacks in unprecedented numbers.

Cancer, too, is related to diet. A recent report from the World Health Organization estimated that about 40 per cent of cancers in men, and a remarkable 60 per cent of cancers in women were linked to diets that had too much fatty food – especially animal fats – and not enough vegetables and fruit. Apart from the links between smoking and lung cancer, diet was the main cause of cancer, especially of the mouth, stomach and bowel, as well as cancers of the breast and womb.

Piles (haemorrhoids) and various other bowel diseases occurring in later life are often the result of a lifetime of eating low-fibre food.

Other diseases are related to eating too much and becoming overweight. Pre-eclampsia, toxaemia and maternal deaths are more common among overweight mothers. Infertility is also related to excess weight. Babies' low birth weights, poor physical condition and congenital defects have been related to the mothers' nutritional status.

From conception to coronaries, cancer to constipation, diet is being recognized as a major factor in our general health. Dietary diseases in total are estimated to be costing the NHS well over £1 billion each year.

— What's this to do with under fives? —

A lot! Firstly, the habits that lead to a bad diet start young. Secondly, so do the dietary diseases themselves.

The early signs of heart disease can be found in the arteries of children as young as one year old. It would be several years before the artery might start to deteriorate, but whereas the first set of teeth will be replaced, a diseased artery may never recover.

The state of children's teeth is shameful. Over half of British children will have tooth decay before their second set of teeth arrive.

Food allergies, particularly allergies to cow's milk and to food additives like the colouring agent tartrazine, have been blamed for asthma, eczema, skin rashes, sleeplessness, hyperactivity and learning problems. Some children with these symptoms have shown an improvement on an additive-free diet, the improvement being greatest for pre-school children.

Habits learned young will be hardest to break. A childhood full of bad eating will increase the chance of serious disease in adulthood. Of a 100 toddlers, 50 will, on current figures, become medically overweight in adulthood, 40 will die of diet-related heart and cardiovascular diseases (ten of them before they reach retirement age), ten will die of diet-related cancers and 90 will have tooth decay by the time they are in their teens. A lot of this suffering can be prevented.

— What can be done? —

Many thousands of children under five benefit from either all-day or sessional nurseries. This means that millions of meals and snacks are given every week to the country's under-fives through day-care facilities.

This book has been designed to give guidance to nursery and catering staff on feeding young children.

— Healthy eating every day —

If it were just a need to get enough vitamins, minerals and other essential nutrients, these could be packaged into a pill for breakfast and there would be no more worry the rest of the day. However, the fact is that most dietary diseases in Britain nowadays are not due to a lack of the right nutrients but to an excess of the wrong ones.

The majority of dietary diseases, particularly common among families on low incomes, are not due to nutrient deficiency but to overconsumption of foods rich in sugar and fat. The main deficiency is simply too little dietary fibre – the 'roughage' provided by fresh fruit and vegetables, wholemeal cereals, pulses, nuts and seeds.

DIETARY GUIDELINES

Many District Health Authorities have introduced food and health policies. These may or may not include advice on feeding young children but it is worth finding out. Contact your local District or Community Dietitian or your local Health Education or Health Promotion Officer. These can all be contacted through your District Hospital.

If advice is unavailable the following guidelines may be of use:-

— Children under one year old —

Infant Feeding Nothing can match breast milk, which can supply all the nutritional needs for the first four to six months of life, gradually changing its composition to meet the needs of the growing baby. It also provides some immunity from infections and diseases and can help prevent allergies or lessen their severity. It may help prevent heart disease in later life. It is, simply, the best food for human babies.

If breast feeding is impossible then commercial infant formula feeds are available. No other sort of milk should be used.

Infant Formula Feeds Most types of formulas are based on cows' milk, and although improved and modified over the years to resemble human milk, formula feeds are still only a distant approximation. The protein is

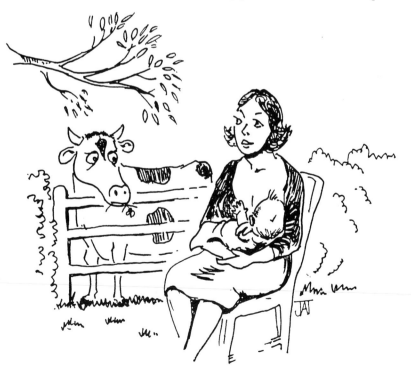

different, there may be more saturated fat and less useful linoleic acid and lipase. Formulas lack the anti-infective and immunological properties of breast milk. Also, of course, they cost money and make work. Some types are based on soya but these should only be used when recommended medically.

No cereals or thickeners should be put in the bottle as they can alter the nutrient balance of the feed, and cause thirst and dehydration. Thinning the formula may underfeed the baby.

Milk Ordinary cows' milk should not be given to babies under the age of six months and preferably not under nine months old as a main milk feed. Start with small quantities, perhaps mixed with potatoes or fish. Giving cows' milk too early may encourage allergies, and the salt levels in cows milk are too high for young kidneys to cope with.

Concern about the danger of saturated fats has led some people to give skimmed milk to babies. Neither the UK Department of Health nor the American Medical Association recommend skimmed or semi-skimmed milk for babies and infants under two years old. If the child is not to be given full-fat milk then care must be taken to ensure that the calories and nutrients they would have obtained in the milk are made up through other foods.

For babies over six months old 'follow on' milks can be used, but these are expensive compared with ordinary cows' milk, and if the baby is on a good mixed diet they are probably of little value.

Children under one year old must be supervised at all times when eating. The National Children's Bureau (NCB) states that

> Babies who are bottle fed should be held and have warm physical contact with an attentive adult whilst being fed. It is strongly recommended that a baby is fed by the same staff member at each feed. Babies should never be left propped up with bottles as it is dangerous and inappropriate to babies' emotional needs.

— Weaning —

The best foods to introduce a baby to are pureed cooked vegetables, fruit, potatoes and other starchy vegetables and ground cereals such as rice or fine cornmeal made into a porridge.

Commercial baby foods may be useful when you are travelling or when you are in a hurry, but they are of poorer quality than freshly cooked meals. Also, children can easily become accustomed to commercial flavours instead of to home cooking. This is fine for food manufacturers, but less good for the long-term health of children.

The first solids are usually introduced between the ages of four and six months, depending on how hungry the baby is. A baby will now need more iron – and other tastes and textures. Weaning develops the chewing mechanism, satisfies increasing appetite and leads gradually to full independence. Food should be given to the baby on a spoon, during or after a breast or bottle feed.

As the baby's appetite grows so can the range of foods. Try blending meat, liver or poultry, fish or lentils. As chewing starts the textures can become coarser and you can gradually try pieces of fruit, sandwiches, toast etc. By one year old the child should be eating the same type of food as the older children (and the staff) in the nursery, although it may still need to be mashed or broken up into small pieces.

The NCB again:

> Parents should always be consulted about when they wish solids to be introduced and which solids to provide. Parents may wish to provide their own baby foods . . . and it is recommended that the nursery not disrupt patterns established at the home.

> Staff should encourage the children to relax while eating and respect the children's preferences and speed of eating, encourage good nutritional habits, and their independence in serving and feeding themselves.

Eggs Introduce these carefully, and not before six old months, as some babies develop an allergy to eggs. Start with the yolks, which are more easily digested than whites – leave whites for another three months or so. All eggs should be cooked until both white and yolk are solid.

Citrus Fruits and Soft Summer Fruits These can also provoke allergic reactions and are not recommended under the age of six months.

Some babies can tolerate a little very diluted orange juice but water and milk are safer.

Wheat The gluten in wheat can provoke intolerance reactions, so wheat-based foods such as cereals and bread are best avoided while the baby is under six months old.

Spinach, Beetroot and Turnip Very rarely these can lead to a certain type of anaemia. You may wish to avoid these until after six months.

Nuts Nuts can provoke allergies in babies under six months old. After this age, finely ground nuts, nut pastes and smooth peanut butter can be given.

Peanut allergy

Although peanut butter is an excellent food for most children and useful in weaning, very occasionally it can provoke severe reactions such as facial swelling and breathing difficulties, which require immediate hospital treatment. Nursery staff need to be aware of this danger and we advise checking with a child's parents before giving peanut butter for the first time.

WEANING – HOW? WHAT? WHY? WHEN?

4–6 months	6–8 months	9–12 months
YOU CAN GIVE:	YOU CAN ADD	YOU CAN ADD
Pureed fruit	A wider range of pureed foods and vegetables	An increasingly wide range of foods with a variety of textures and flavours
Pureed vegetables	Purees which include chicken, fish and liver	Cows' milk
Thin porridge made from oat or rice flakes or cornmeal	Wheat-based foods, e.g. mashed Weetabix	Pieces of cheese
Finely pureed dhal or lentils	Egg-yolk, well cooked	Fromage frais
	Small-sized beans such as aduki beans, cooked soft	Yogurt
HOW:	Pieces of ripe banana	Pieces of fish
Offer the food on the tip of a clean finger or on the tip of a clean (plastic or horn) teaspoon	Cooked rice	Soft cooked beans
	Citrus fruits	Smooth peanut butter
	Soft summer fruits	Pasta
	Pieces of bread	A variety of breads
WHEN:		Pieces of meat from a casserole
A very tiny amount at first, during or after a milk feed	HOW	Well-cooked egg white
	On a teaspoon	Or almost anything that is wholesome and that the child can swallow
WHY:		
The start of transition from milk to solids	WHEN	HOW
	At the end of a milk feed	On a spoon or as finger food
NOT YET:		
Cows' milk – or any except breast or formula milk	WHY	WHY
Citrus fruit	To introduce other foods when the child is hungry	To encourage full independence
Soft summer fruits		
Wheat (cereals, flour, bread etc.)	NOT YET	NOT YET
Spices	Cows' milk, except in small quantities mixed with other food	Whole nuts
Spinach, swede, turnip, beetroot	Chillies or chilli powder (e.g. cayenne)	Salt
Eggs	Egg whites	Sugar
Nuts	Nuts	Fatty food
Salt	Salt	
Sugar	Sugar	
Fatty food	Fatty food	

Salt No salt should be added to weaning foods. Babies' kidneys cannot cope with it.

Spices Most spices and herbs are tolerated well in weaning foods, but chillies and chilli powder can cause upsets in some children.

Sugar Adding extra sugar to babyfood may damage new teeth and will encourage a 'sweet tooth'. Sugar provides calories without any nutrients - empty calories. If you buy ready-made foods look for sorts without any sugar: check the ingredients list to avoid sugar in various forms: sucrose, glucose, dextrose, fructose, maltose, syrup, honey, 'raw' or brown sugar, or concentrated fruit juice. Look for sugar in medicines and see if there is a sugar-free version - there is of Calpol, for example, but you have to ask for it.

Allergies to such things as eggs, wheat, citrus and soft summer fruits, afflict only a small number of children, but you should be aware of the possibility. Be particularly careful with children from families with a history of allergy.

How to puree food

USE:

A fork to mash soft foods, e.g. banana, potato

A sieve and a large spoon or possibly the end of a *very* well-scrubbed (handle-less!) rolling pin for larger amounts

A rotary whisk or hand-held blender

A potato masher

A Mouli-sieve – not very well known in Britain, but available and cheap. It will sieve quite stiff mixtures in no time, leaving behind skins and seeds. Comes with three different bases to give three different textures from fine to coarse

A liquidiser (or food processor for larger amounts) which will puree almost anything – skins, seeds and all

---

Additives Certain additives are banned from baby foods but others, such as flavourings, are permitted even though they have no nutritional value. Other foods, such as soft drinks, snack foods and sweets, have a wide range of additives. These are of no value to babies, and they will not help babies to learn about real food and may even provoke allergies and behaviour problems. (Read pages 9–10 on additives.)

Pulses and Dhals (split pulses) Dhals can be introduced as a weaning food from about four months as long as they are smooth. Well-cooked, mashed small beans such as mung and aduki beans are suitable from about six to eight months and larger beans such as well-cooked kidney beans and chickpeas can be introduced a few months later.

Vitamins Most children eating a well-balanced varied diet will not need vitamin supplements. However, the Department of Health advises that all children under the age of two years and preferably until five years old should receive special supplements of vitamins A, C and D in the form of drops which are available from the local child health clinic or Health Visitors.

Dietary fibre It is only in the last few generations that human beings have eaten refined white flour, rice, pasta and the like. Natural whole grains are preferable to their refined counterparts as they have more nutrients and useful dietary fibre. However, one must note that:

1   A sudden change to a more whole-grain diet can lead to excessive bowel movements — a phase that could last for several weeks until the digestive system has adjusted. A gradual change is essential.
2   Bran (the fibre found in whole grains of wheat and oats) should not be added to foods for the same reason. Also, too much pure bran in the diet can absorb and remove nutrients.

As well as whole grains, all fruits, especially peaches and strawberries, and all vegetables, especially parsnips, potatoes, plantains, sweetcorn, lentils, beans and even frozen peas are good sources of fibre.
Laxatives should not be needed when the diet has enough fibre.

— Children one to five years old —

Milk Milk provides many useful nutrients. An average of a pint a day is usually recommended for children under the age of five. More than two pints can limit the appetite for other essential foods.
There has been some debate about the type of milk children under five should be drinking: skimmed, semi-skimmed or full-fat. There is growing evidence that fat in the diet in childhood is related to heart disease later in life, and that saturated fats in particular are responsible. Full-fat milk is a major source of saturated fats in many children's diets. On the other hand, full-fat milk has more calories and has vitamins A and D, useful for children whose diet is otherwise poor.
If children are eating a good range of foods then semi-skimmed milk may seem a good compromise. If you want more advice then contact your District Hospital's dietetic department.

Fats The strongest evidence relating fat intake to heart disease is for saturated fats. Cutting back dramatically on all fat may lead to problems in getting enough calories in the diet. It may be better to cut down on the saturated fats rather than all fats. This could be achieved by reducing the amount of fatty meats and meat products, butter, cheese, lard and hard margarine. Use more fish and lean meats, and use margarines and oils based on corn, sunflower or soya.

Sugar There is little doubt that sugar intake in children is related to tooth decay. Sugar provides no nutrients other than calories, and it is often associated with fat in the food, e.g. in cakes and biscuits. Diets containing a lot of sugar may also be relatively low in vitamins, minerals and fibre.

Sugar itself is unnecessary as a source of energy. All starchy foods are digested to form glucose which is the body's main energy source. Brown sugar and honey, which are just as bad for teeth, contain only insignificant amounts of minerals.

Dietary Fibre With less fat and sugar in the diet, the child is more likely to be eating starchy and bulky food such as bread, potatoes, rice, pasta, fruit and vegetables. The child's stomach can fill up with this bulk even though he or she hasn't actually had enough calories to last until the next main meal. In such circumstances, between-meal snacks such as fruit, dried fruit, sandwiches and the like, become of increasing importance.

In a well-balanced diet the specially concentrated sources of fibre such as bran are not necessary and should not be given unless specifically prescribed.

Salt By the time a child is over a year old there should be little risk of kidney damage from excess salt. However, current evidence suggests that there may be a link between high salt intakes and high blood pressure in later life. It is sensible that children do not develop a taste for highly salted foods and so it is better if little or no salt is used in preparing and cooking foods. Remember not to cook vegetables in salted water: the salt is quite unnecessary and the cooking water will be too salty to use for anything else. Vegetable cooking water can be tasty and nutritious in stews and soups, but keep it in the fridge and use within a day.

Salt-shakers should never be put on children's meal tables – indeed they need not exist in the nursery at all.

Nuts It is recommended that children under the age of five should not be given whole nuts. There is a possible danger of choking and there are further complications from inhaling a piece of nut which do not result from inhaling most other foods. Nuts are a good source of unsaturated fats, protein and B vitamins, so peanut butter (and other nut pastes) are a useful alternative – look for ones without added sweeteners, salt or other fats or oils.

— Additives —

Most additives are used only to make food seem more attractive than it would be without the additives. They are 'cosmetics' for the food – the colours, flavourings, texturizers, flavour enhancers, bulking agents, emulsifiers, and even the preservatives and anti-oxidants, which keep the food looking fresh and germ-free when it is months old. So a long list of 'E' numbers might make you suspicious about how fresh and wholesome the food really is.

Government food regulations advise against certain additives in food meant specifically for babies and young children, including artificial sweeteners like saccharin and NutraSweet, some preservatives and some flavour enhancers like monosodium glutamate. But a lot of food that children eat, whether crisps or orange squash, raisins or ice lollies, is not sold as being 'specifically for babies and young children' and so may contain the full range of additives.

Children with suspected food-related problems including asthma, eczema, skin rashes or hyperactivity should seek medical advice, and may be advised to avoid many of the following list of suspect additives:

Colourings (azo dyes)

E102 tartrazine
E104 quinoline yellow
E107 yellow 2G
E110 sunset yellow
E122 carmiosine
E123 amaranth
E124 ponceau
E128 red 2G
E131 patent blue
E132 indigo carmine
 133 brilliant blue
E142 green S
E151 black PN
 154 brown FK
 155 brown HT
E180 pigment rubine

Colours (others)

E127   erythrosine
E150   caramels
E160b solvent extracted annatto
E161g canthaxanthin

Preservatives

Benzoates: E210–E219
Sulphites: E220–E224, E226, E227
Nitrates/nitrites: E249, E250, E251, E252
Anti-oxidant gallates: E310, E311, E312
Anti-oxidants BHA and BHT: E320, E321

Sweeteners and flavour enhancers

Aspartame, saccharin
Monosodium glutamate: 621

— Meat —

Decades of poor animal husbandry have produced increasing numbers of unhealthy animals and, as a result, meat and eggs which are frequently infected with food poisoning bacteria. Great care must be taken to cook all meat and eggs thoroughly in order to destroy any dangerous bacteria they may contain. (For more on food hygiene, see Chapter five.)

CHAPTER TWO

Changing for the Better

In summary, children are eating:

- Too much sugar
- Too much salt
- Too much fat
- Too much refined white starch
- Too many additives and processed foods
- Too few fresh fruits and vegetables

So what can we do?

1   Cut down on ready-prepared foods and drinks that contain sugar. Avoid recipes which need sugar or, at least, cut the amount of sugar called for by half, or sweeten with banana or dried fruits.
2   Cut down on ready-prepared foods that are salty. Cook vegetables in unsalted water – and save the water. Use the merest speck of salt to flavour dishes – or use none at all.
3   Avoid ready-prepared composite dishes – burgers, sausages, pies etc. Cut down on chips (try the oven chips on page 140). Avoid using much red meat and cut off all visible fat. Use good, named oils (e.g. sunflower, corn) and polyunsaturated spreads.
4   Avoid ready-made white flour products – cakes, pies, bread, buns. Cook with either wholemeal flour (100% of the grain) or 'wheatmeal' flour (80%). Use brown rice, brown pasta (looks much lighter when cooked!), brown semolina, pot barley, oats.
5   Avoid packet puddings and toppings, which are mostly made of sugar, starch and additives.
6   Eat more fresh produce.
7   For the sake of hygiene, cook all meat, poultry and eggs really thoroughly.
8   Try vegetarian dishes.
9   Try fish dishes.

— But they LIKE chips and burgers! —

Of course! They've been fed them often enough to develop a taste for them! And, of course, these foods seem juicy and succulent, but that is mainly *because* of the large amount of fat in them. A child cannot possibly be expected to understand the damage these foods are doing, but we can – and must – if we are to protect the children in our care: we must seize every opportunity to educate children's taste buds *away* from the tempting but salty, fatty foods so universally available and *towards* the flavours of healthy cooking. But how best to go about it?

A few tips:

1 Make changes slowly and unobtrusively. One change at a time
2 Accustom children to a wide range of foods early on
3 Create fun activities involving food
4 Presentation – make the food *look* delicious
5 Be seen to eat it yourself with obvious pleasure
6 Explain briefly why you are making changes, if asked
7 Give 'good' foods as treats, not 'bad' ones
8 Be absolutely positive in your approach

AND DON'T ever say 'Eat it up, it will do you good!'

And now, in more detail:

—— HOW TO GO ABOUT MAKING CHANGES ——

Make changes slowly

Most children – and adults too – prefer familiar well-liked food to some unfamiliar food which is an unknown quantity.

A sudden withdrawal of old favourites and substitution of strange new things could seem like a punishment, and you could be lost almost before you've started. Sweeping changes in food, as in anything else, often create feelings of insecurity and a demand to return to the original state, so avoid this kind of defeat by spreading the changes over many weeks. Rather than banning, say, commercial beefburgers once and for all, start by having them a bit less often, then just occasionally, and eventually, perhaps after five or six months, they can disappear almost imperceptibly.

Some changes, such as to brown rice or brown pasta from white, will hardly be noticed as, once cooked, both colour and texture are quite similar, but the difference between wholemeal bread and white is much more noticeable. Go slowly here: at first, change *occasionally* to a brown-looking and soft-crusted loaf (such as granary, Vit-B Wheatgerm or Hovis) and wait until the children have completely accepted that before gradually introducing real wholemeal. It's often a good strategy to serve a permanent mixture of many different kinds of bread, so that bread becomes a thing of interest in itself. Try flat Greek loaves, pitta, nan, chapatis, French sticks, rye bread – whatever you can get.

Be guided by the children: they will let you know whether they are enjoying the novelty of new tastes or whether it's time to pull back for a while. Letting them play with a new food first (see chapter 7) often works wonders.

Give a wide range of foods early on

We know that food preferences are usually established before the age of five. Use the pre-school years well by making food a varied and interesting, even exciting, experience. We now have the greatest variety of foods from all over the world that we have ever had on sale – what a pity to ignore them and just serve the same boring mass-produced stuff over and over! Pimentos, garlic, mushrooms, mangoes are all suitable foods for young children and no more 'exotic' than potatoes or oranges after all.

Work to avoid the 'Don't-like-it-never-had-it' syndrome. Present new foods often, at fairly well-spaced out intervals and, at least at first, in small quantities or as a choice item.

Present a new food as an activity item

Try introducing foods in the context of 'This is fun!' rather than 'Oh dear, have I got to eat this funny-looking stuff'. For example, show a big turnip before telling 'The Tale of the Turnip' and at the end say that if we're *very lucky*, the cook might be able to make it into turnip soup for tomorrow's dinner. What colour do you think the soup would be? Brown? Red? Cut the turnip open (turnips are *hard*) and guess again. (Turnip soup is almost pure white and amazingly good, see the recipe on page 129.) Remind the children the next morning that there's going to be that special turnip soup – cook has managed it! Wasn't that kind? We must thank her very much for cooking our story-turnip. And so on . . . (Read Chapters 7–10 for more ideas.)

Presentation: sounding and looking good

Will children actually eat the healthy food, when they know they could always scream for cakes, puddings, sweets? The answer is yes, but it may require some imagination. A lot depends on *presentation*. A good idea is to take a look at what food companies do – what tricks have they used to make their products look attractive to children? Try mixtures of colours, unusual shapes, various textures, attractive wrappings, funny names: 'baby' carrots, 'monster' pie, 'green trees' (broccoli), 'white trees' (cauliflorets), 'pipes' (macaroni), or themes involving animals, dolls, magic, a favourite song or story as above. If turnip soup is popular it could go into the repertoire – 'Story-Turnip Soup'. What's in a name? A very great deal! We have known a liver casserole described as 'wolf stew' to be eaten amazingly eagerly. 'Snowball Pudding', 'Funny-Face Fish,' 'the Giant's Special Beanstalk Stew' just *sound* inviting – even without one's having the least idea what they are!

Colour is vital – mashed potato, cauliflower and white sauce on a white plate even *sounds* awful, but it's so easy to forget and dish up such a thing.

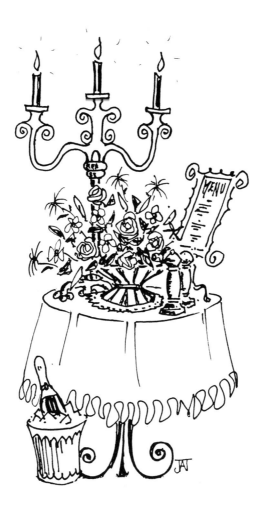

A lot depends on presentation.

The white turnip soup in a brown earthenware casserole dish served into little coloured bowls, and/or garnished with finely cut carrot sticks is the general idea. And yes, *garnish* is as important for children as for anyone else! Even just a quick scattering of fresh chopped parsley or a dusting of paprika can make all the difference.

Save and use celery leaves, chopped spring onion tops, chopped watercress stalks as 'free' garnishes. Small pieces of curly kale in winter are a cheap garnish – one head will do a week's garnishes, if wrapped in damp paper inside a plastic bag in the fridge. The rest of it can go into soup – such as the minestrone recipe on page 128.

'To be acceptable, children's food should be varied, even a little startling and pretty enough to please the eye. I am all for the flower in the fish's mouth, the daisy in the salad,' writes Molly Keane in her delightful 'Nursery Cooking.' How true!

Consider too, the colour scheme of the eating area as a whole. Think about, especially when re-ordering equipment, the colour of the plates in relation to the colour of the beakers, the tables or tablecovers – see the whole scene. Are there two or three flowers in a sturdy pot on each table, nasturtiums, marigolds, pinks, catmint, perhaps from the nursery garden? All easy to grow; maybe with a sprig of rosemary or thyme, or have just a few daisies, buttercups or grasses in flower. In winter, have bulbs in pots or displaying their roots in glass jars which can be put on the tables at meal time, or silvery honesty sprays. Or at least have good postcard photographs of flowers mounted on stiff card, tied at the top in pairs and leaning back to back.

Table cloths look better than formica: use any pretty cotton fabric cut to size and over the top lay a piece of plain translucent plastic to cover completely. Or use an attractive PVC-coated fabric. If you keep the overhang short, there should be little problem with pulling.

Or, you may prefer place-mats, and some nurseries have little cotton napkins, all washed out at the end of each day, and which the children soon learn to use. It depends on your situation – customs vary.

Such things as flowers and table-coverings are only a little more trouble and do help enormously to achieve a less institutional atmosphere, and also somehow to say 'Now it's dinner time: play is over for the moment. This is our (comparatively) quiet, enjoyable eating time'.

Eat it yourself

Good food is good food – whether for children or adults. Sugar is particularly dangerous for children's teeth but it will rot teeth of any age. Not only is it a tremendous bonus for nursery staff to be able to have the same nutritious fare as the children, but it is also important for the children to feel that adults do eat the same things as they do, and with obvious enjoyment. Sardines on toast must be all right because you eat them too. In fact this is a very effective way of encouraging young children to accept unfamiliar food.

(If you feel you need a little push yourself in the direction of a healthier diet – here is the opportunity!)

If asked, tell

From time to time, you will probably be asked about some of the changes you are making. Have your replies ready, so you're not left with something as lame as 'Well, it's better for you'. On the one hand, you can say that 'brown' bread is tastier than white and that there's more to chew, or that oranges/pears/satsumas are so nice and fresh and juicy to eat at the end of a meal or, in the summer, frying chips makes the kitchen too hot; or that those ready-prepared desserts are too expensive now; or that cooking a pudding every day is hard work, and it's kind if we don't ask cook to do that too often; or that yogurt tastes so clean and fresh and cool – like snow! And so on.

On the other hand, it is perfectly possible to tell a brief and simplified version of the truth about your overall strategy. Say, truthfully, that sugar makes teeth go brown and black and can make you have awful toothache, so it's really rather unkind to keep giving food with sugar in it to people. Or you could say that all those chips/burgers/sausages etc. are too greasy (or fatty or oily). Greasy food makes your blood too thick and sticky and that can stop your body working properly and make you very ill and, again, it's not really fair to give a lot of greasy food to people for them to eat.

Just a *little bit, sometimes*, you should add, before the children think they'll never see chips or custard again in the nursery and develop an instant yearning for them.

That certain foods can make you ill is a truth: there is no reason why this truth should not be (suitably) told to young children in what is, after all, an educational establishment.

Give high quality a high profile!

Make treats high quality. It really is extraordinary how, whenever a child is given an edible treat, it is probably something quite unhealthy! Reverse this by giving foods that are both delicious *and* nutritious — pieces of mango or nectarine, sweet seedless grapes, halved plums, big golden gooseberries, strawberries, raspberries, red-currants 'because they are so delicious and we don't often have them'. Don't forget to give savoury foods as a treat too: perhaps thin slices of cheese with fruit bread, cheese scones or rolls, wedges of an excellent pizza, halves of small filled jacket potatoes, perhaps a favourite item on toast. . .

If there is something you are trying to 'push,' making it the 'treat' item can prove effective: carrots *must* be something rather good if they're served (say, as cruditées) as party food! As for the practice of giving a sweet as a spontaneous reward or encouragement, well, grazed knees and bumped heads are not 'made better,' nor do children feel specially rewarded by the offer of a sweet or such *unless* things have been set up like that.

Expressions of warm feeling – exclamations of praise, a special hug – are to be preferred to encouraging a habit that leads inexorably to the dentist's drill.

If you want to give something tangible, a coloured paper star or just a square of paper with a smiley face quickly drawn on it and stuck with tape onto the child's jumper will seem *exactly* as desirable – *if* that is your established custom. It will last longer, too, and can be shown off at home.

Of course, the attitude of staff in all this, as in anything else, is crucial. An adult who doesn't like (or is unused to) wholemeal bread or fresh fish, may have to put on a brave face! Just one observed grimace and a good new dish may be doomed before it's even tasted.

Be positive

Your desire for good food should be as serious and as professional as it is for good play equipment and good books. Become an expert on the benefits of good food and the dangers of bad. Perhaps start with the books on the reading list (page 156). The more knowledge you have the easier it will be to make the right decisions – and stick to your guns!

— And a reminder... —

Saying 'Eat-it-up-it-will-do-you-good' makes food sound like medicine. Let them see *you* tucking in!

CHAPTER THREE
What's for Dinner?

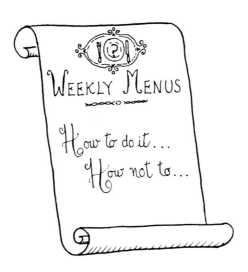

We have said that changing to a really healthy way of eating can take time because it is best done very gradually. There must be a certain level of commitment on the part of staff and it is marvellous if you also catch the imagination of the children's parents or carers. You may find it helpful to have a meeting with them fairly early on to explain what you're trying to do and why. Their interest and support can make the world of difference.

Your weekly menus may not look that much different for a few weeks – one less sugary pudding per week, chips slightly less often, occasionally a different kind of bread . . . but your aim is to carry the children with you – *and* the staff and parents.

Whatever you give the children, they should *enjoy* it, whatever stage of change you have got to. If your particular children simply adore sausages and are always asking when they are going to have sausages again, it would be foolish – and downright unkind – to say 'Never'. In fact you might decide that sausages would be the very last food to be removed from your 'undesirable' list, or even still have them very occasionally. You might decide, of course, to serve them with potatoes in their jackets instead of chips; you also may find that sausages eventually cease to be such a favourite as against some of the new dishes coming onto the menu.

Perhaps a local butcher would make you a batch of sausages with less fat and salt and no dye or preservative? Some butchers will do this. Collect and cook (or freeze) the sausages the same day. Roast the sausages in a covered pan in the oven for about an hour, at gas 4, 350°F, 165°C, or until well cooked.

However, you do need a goal in mind, so here are two suggested weekly menus, both served successfully by a nursery in London, and, by contrast, another type of menu, probably all too familiar to many nursery staff.

A WEEK'S MENU IN A LONDON NURSERY

The kitchen is on the premises.

This nursery provides a lunch-time meal, drinks at 4pm and then a tea-time snack for children staying on after 4.30 p.m. Water is always served with dinner.

Week I

Monday	12.00	Lentil casserole
		Side salad (lettuce, carrot, cucumber)
		Plain yogurt with bananas
	4.30 p.m.	Vegetarian samosas
		Milk
Tuesday	12.00	Tuna risotto
		Fresh fruit
	4.30 p.m.	Wholewheat crackers
		Cottage cheese
		Fresh apple juice, diluted
Wednesday	12.00	Haddock hot-pot
		Fresh carrots and runner beans
		Stewed apple and natural yogurt
	4.30 p.m.	Cold chicken pieces, wholemeal crackers
		Fruit juice, diluted
Thursday	12.00	Vegetarian curry and rice
		Plain yogurt with oranges
	4.30 p.m.	Wholemeal pasties (root vegetables and haricot beans)
		Milk
Friday	12.00	West-Indian chicken
		Rice and peas
		Cheese and biscuits
	4.30 p.m.	Wholemeal baps
		Egg mayonnaise
		Fruit juice, diluted

— So what's so good about this one? —

A lot of things! Here are some of them:

- Whole grain bread and crackers, not white
- Fresh fruit or real fruit juice every day – not the synthetic or sugared kinds
- Lots of vegetables every day
- Plain, unsugared yogurt three times during the week, not the commercial ones with low (or imitation) fruit and high sugar.
- Fish twice in the week, without resorting to expensive fish fingers, and including tuna, an extra-beneficial oily fish.
- No sugar or sugar substitutes at all
- Nothing, except the tuna, out of a tin
- Only two recipes that involve frying
- Dishes from a variety of countries
- Home cooking!
- It *sounds* attractive

SECOND WEEK'S MENUS IN A LONDON NURSERY

Week 2

Monday	12.00	Vegetable broth Macaroni cheese Fresh tomatoes and jacket potatoes
	4.30 p.m.	Hummus and carrot sandwiches Fresh apple juice, diluted
Tuesday	12.00	Fillet of whiting stuffed with prawns, with Mornay sauce Fresh mangos
	4.30 p.m.	Boiled eggs Bread and butter Milk
Wednesday	12.00	Kedgeree Natural yogurt
	4.30 p.m.	Chinese spring rolls Carrot juice, diluted
Thursday	12.00	Tuna and courgette wholewheat flan Sweetcorn and green salad Plain yogurt with fresh, stoned cherries
	4.30 p.m.	Wholemeal pizza slices Home-made lemonade
Friday	12.00	Chilli con carne and rice Wholemeal apricot crumble
	4.30 p.m.	Onion bhajis Hot chocolate

— Or this? —

The same kind of things! In general terms, both weeks' menus use only nutritious foods. Old adages like 'Eat a balanced diet,' and 'Eat a variety of foods,' may be good in theory, but are quite unhelpful in menu planning. It's not enough to say 'Every meal should contain some carbohydrate.' What *type* of carbohydrate? There's a world of difference between a wholemeal bap and a doughnut! We must say *wholegrain* – and no sugar added. And that terrible old cliché 'Everything in moderation', is as untruthful now as it ever was: indeed, nursery children should *not* be given fatty meat or sugary dessert toppings in moderation – or at all, while wholewheat bread can be eaten at will.

The modern 'Balanced Diet' means planning menus of good, nutritious food, not padded out with anything else, thus:

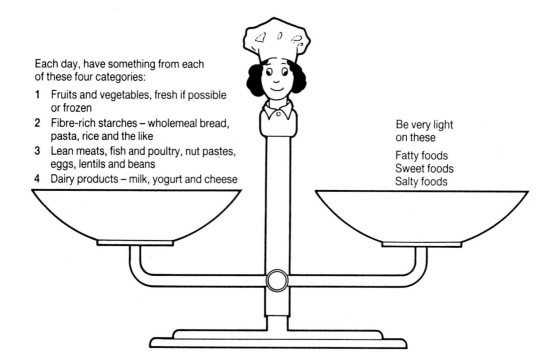

Each day, have something from each
of these four categories:

1 Fruits and vegetables, fresh if possible
   or frozen
2 Fibre-rich starches – wholemeal bread,
   pasta, rice and the like
3 Lean meats, fish and poultry, nut pastes,
   eggs, lentils and beans
4 Dairy products – milk, yogurt and cheese

Be very light
on these

Fatty foods
Sweet foods
Salty foods

The skill of cooking means combining and presenting these foods in a delicious and visually attractive way, day after day.

LIMIT	TRY
Frying/deep frying	Stir-frying, grilling
Roasting in fat	Baking or steaming
Adding salt	Adding herbs/spices
Serving fat and skin on meat	Skimming fat off stews gravy, etc.
Hard fats (butter, ghee, palm or coconut oil, lard)	Sunflower, corn, soya, olive oils
White flour	Wholegrain flour
White rice	Brown rice
Over-cooking vegetables or letting them stand around	Raw vegetables, or ones cooked quickly
Sugar in recipes	Substitute dried fruit

— Breakfast —

If your nursery offers breakfast, you could serve a similar breakfast each day, such as:

BREAKFAST MENU

A wholewheat cereal (shredded wheat, puffed wheat, Weetabix) or a sugar-free muesli base, perhaps cooked)
Wholemeal toast;
Fresh orange juice.

You can make you own cereal from crumbled wholewheat or granary bread, toasted. Add hot or cold milk and perhaps a pinch of cinnamon.

— And so what's wrong with this menu? —

Monday	Lunch	Toad in the hole
		Mashed swede
		Roast potatoes
	Dessert	Suet pudding
		Custard
	Tea	Hamburgers
		Tomatoes
		Chips
Tuesday	Lunch	Fried bacon
		Cabbage
		Mashed potatoes
	Dessert	Tapioca pudding
		Jam
	Tea	Roast chicken legs (cold)
		Tomatoes and cucumber salad
Wednesday	Lunch	Cheese and egg flan
		Cauliflower
		Chips
	Dessert	Apple fritters
		Ice cream
	Tea	Sausage rolls
		Baked beans
Thursday	Lunch	Meat pie
		Mashed potatoes
		Tinned spaghetti
		Sweetcorn
	Dessert	Tinned fruit salad
		Condensed milk
	Tea	Jam sandwiches
		Crisps
Friday	Lunch	Fish fingers
		Spaghetti hoops
		Fried potatoes
	Dessert	Treacle tart
		Custard
	Tea	Fried egg
		Peas
		Chips

How many mistakes can you find?
Then turn over...

— The long list of lost opportunities —

- No whole grains – just lots of refined white, low-fibre starch.
- Not just one, but *two* sugary dessert items every single day.
- No fresh fruit at all
- A green vegetable only twice
- No yogurt at all
- No pulses – except tinned (i.e. sugared and salted) baked beans.
- Heavy quantities of fat at every meal
- Fish only once and no fresh fish. No oily fish
- A total of ten foods that are fried!
- Ready-made commercial foods used, which means lots of fat, salt and additives
- Enormous amounts of calories from fats, sugar and starch, but yielding comparatively small amounts of nutrients
- No provision for children of other cultures
- Every meal heavy, fatty, low fibre, high salt and high sugar!
- Too much work for a Friday. Not workable.

Two particular points

1 **The jam sandwich** Jam eaten together with white bread is very damaging for teeth. The fine white flour in the bread mixes with saliva to form a sticky paste. This paste, mixed with the sugar in the jam, sticks onto the teeth, holding the sugar in place to eat away at the precious tooth enamel.

2 **Tinned fruit salad and condensed milk** Why *ever* not fresh fruit? The tinned sort is saturated with thick syrup, and probably served with it, too. Condensed milk is sweetened. Evaporated would have been better as it isn't, or yogurt.

Children like simple food. The food in these menus is too overpowering, too 'cooked up'.

— Gaining the bad, losing the good —

Menus like this make children lose out twice:

- *Once* because of the huge overconsumption of sugar, salt and fat – leading to the diseases so prevalent in Britain like tooth decay, obesity, heart disease, diabetes, strokes, etc.
- *And again* because of the nutritious and beneficial food that *could* have been eaten instead of the damaging food. The child has, for example, had all that fat and sugar and vast numbers of calories in the apple

fritters and ice cream, and not had the vitamin C and the fibre and mouth-cleansing effect that, say, half a raw apple would have provided.

— A word on salads —

Salads are great but they take up a lot of stomach space. Accompany or follow a salad with something more filling, or be ready to serve a healthy snack after a while. Beware of confusing the needs of an adult who might be trying to slim, with the quite different needs of a growing child.

—————— AND WHAT OF SNACKS THEN? ——————

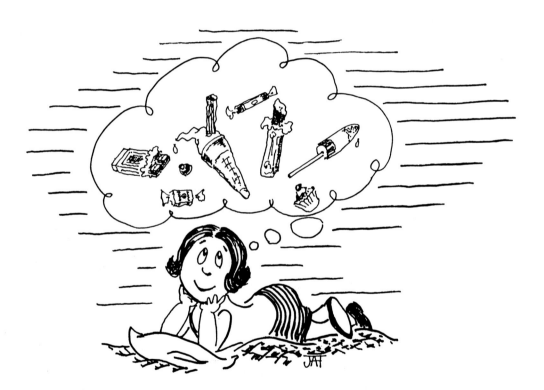

Yes, some children really need snacks! But . . . no, not like the above.

The thing is, children's stomachs are small – they fill up quickly and empty quickly. Babies need feeding many times a day; adults go about five hours between their 'Three square meals a day'. Young children are somewhere between the two. Three 'proper' meals with maybe up to three 'mini' meals in between are needed by some children.

The trick is to feed children when they are hungry whilst giving them something that you can completely justify nutritionally. *Never* give anything sugary as a snack because sugar is an appetite depressant and could well spoil the child's appetite for the next meal; and never give anything too fatty – fat takes a long time to digest and again could prevent the child feeling ready for the next meal.

HEALTHIER SNACK IDEAS

- Sandwiches, or rolls, or pitta, filled with peanut butter, tahini, fromage frais, cottage cheese, mashed or sliced banana, cheese or sardines with salad items
- Pieces of fruit: banana, pear, apple, satsumas
- Dried fruit, such as raisins, apricots or apple rings
- Milk or home-made milkshakes (see page 142)
- Pure fruit juices diluted with water
- Sticks of scrubbed carrot, celeriac, parsnip, courgette or celery
- Wholewheat, rye, oat or rice crackers
- Home-made soup.

Some nurseries allow children to bring their own snacks. Fine, if this suits you, but say 'fresh fruit only'. Return anything else with a (courteous) reminder.

—— SOME PSYCHOLOGICAL CONSIDERATIONS ——

It may sound surprising, but food is believed to do you more good if you are happy and relaxed while you are eating it.

Conversely, if you eat whilst angry, anxious or unhappy in any way, the food may be poorly digested and therefore less beneficial.

Nursery dinner time

Long tables seating perhaps a dozen or more, lines of children queuing for toileting, hand-washing, first course, second course, more hand-washing. . . these procedures all work against the relaxed, informal family atmosphere that should be your aim.

Every nursery is different, but it is important to eradicate the queue system as much at meal times as at any other.

One nursery we know changed to a 'key-worker' system many years ago and found it most beneficial. At lunch time, several small tables were laid in each room with a key-worker and the children for whom she was particularly responsible at each one. This encouraged language and sociable interaction between children and staff and enabled the staff to really get to know the children's likes and dislikes and eating difficulties in much more detail. (Also, the children could *see* the adults eating the carrot sticks!) Before and after the meal, each group was more able to move through the toileting and washing routine as a group rather than as a mass.

This one change has provided noticeably better care and understanding between staff and child, particularly with children on the special needs register.

At first, extra washing up was created because each little table had its own bowls of food from which the children helped themselves – important if children were to learn how to select and choose their own amounts of food. However, this was remedied by a review of the type of food served. Instead of the ubiquitous meat, potato and other vegetables all needing separate cooking and serving utensils, newer items on the menu reflecting a multicultural approach (see Chapter 5) were found to require fewer kitchen pots and serving bowls. Having fresh fruit for dessert instead of the previous 'pudding-and-custard' eliminated a huge amount of work – less cooking to do, and fewer cooking pots, less cutlery and both fewer and easier dessert plates to wash up. Finger foods generally – fruit, vegetable sticks, cheese and biscuits or bread, chicken drumsticks, samosas, Mexican tacos – greatly cut down on work.

—— Nursery teatime ——

Serving a 3 o'clock tea-time meal is a common practice in most day nurseries. But quite a few children need a sleep in the afternoon too, and after all the toileting, washing, clearing up and dressing involved with sleep and a second sit-down meal, a child needing sleep can be left with only about 30 minutes' play in the whole afternoon!

One nursery, after much discussion with staff and, most importantly, with parents, abolished the formal, sit-down meal at 3 p.m. Instead, play activities continued and at 3 o'clock, drinks were offered for the children to consume at whatever activity they were doing, whether on the mat with a floor puzzle or at the painting easel (a small chair by the side proved useful for the drink). Spillage was not found to be a problem, the children were free to continue with their chosen activities, to drink at their own pace, alone or with company and, indeed, to decide whether to drink at all.

Many children were collected by 4 pm. Those who remained after 4.30 p.m. were provided with a meal in small, family-type groups, perhaps sitting on the carpet, eating with their fingers, often without plates. This may sound unhygienic compared with the mass hand-washing and formal sit-down tea, but it was thought to be so much more pleasant and home-like – and also realistic. How many children, or adults, sit at a table to eat a sandwich or have a drink? One might consider the rigorous institutionalized hand-washing and formal eating in the nursery in relation to ordinary home life.

This is what one nursery (Nunhead, in Peckham) told us:

Previous to change, many parents had discussed at their child's nursery review (of which they are part) the concern over how little their child ate after being at nursery all day.

It was of concern to know that they were frustrated and angry not to have a meal eaten that they had taken the time to prepare.

Explaining that the children had had a good lunch and tea did not help all the parents.

Over a period of time it became obvious that many parents wanted to give their child food on returning from nursery. I use the word 'food' and not 'meal' because a parent's expression of caring did not have to be in the traditional concept of a meat, potato and vegetable meal: sandwiches, hot snacks etc. were often what the child wanted or what the parent wished to serve.

The main point was that both parent, child and perhaps a family unit, had a chance to share food which brings together a social setting.

One parent explained she felt guilty about working, although she enjoyed it and found it benefited both her and her child. What the parent felt was a loss on her part of caring for the child. Preparing food for the evening was part of the care that was missing.

In day nurseries there may be families that bring extra concerns on whether the children are being fed enough at home.

At Nunhead nursery there was such a family and I was concerned that, not having tea would be detrimental to them. However, it is presumptuous of professional workers to feel that we are the ones that are enabling this family to survive by feeding their children for them.

As a social worker quite rightly said, 'If we give too many supports at this stage, what happens when the child attends school? Schools do not provide tea.'

— Involving parents —

We really cannot emphasize enough just how much your parents should be involved in discussions about making changes *before* they occur.

Once the nursery staff, and in particular the cook herself, are enthusiastic about getting away from the meat-gravy-potatoes-vegetables-pudding-and-custard routine, there will have to be some good discussion and planning ahead. Who, for example, constructs the nursery menus? Although the cook will have to arrange the food orders, it would be a good idea if she could share meal planning with all the staff – and students! A weekly meeting between the cook and nursery head should ensure the smooth running of food budgetting and planning.

We suggest that after the staff have agreed to have a trial of the new regime, you send a letter, such as the following, which was sent out by Nunhead nursery in London:

'Dear Parents,

We have been increasingly concerned about the type of food we offer here and the way it is cooked.

In a few weeks time we will be changing our menu in many aspects. The care staff and our cook, Mrs Balmforth, would like your opinions and welcome discussions on the changes.

What are the changes? Only wholemeal flour, pasta and bread will be used and the children will shop with the staff for various fresh fish and fruit and vegetables that they may not have tasted, such as mango and kohlrabi.

Crisps, sweets, cake and sweet puddings will be discouraged and will not be a constant sight on our Menu Board. Likewise, we will be very discriminating on the use of frozen food. Orange squash also contains a lot of artificial flavours and colour and large amounts of sugar in some brands. Therefore, we will not be using orange squash in the nursery.

Food from other cultures will be included on a regular basis as will fresh salads, fruit and vegetables.

We hope you will be pleased with the changes and make a point of looking on the Menu board. Thank you. '

According to Helen Strange, Officer in Charge:

The letter was received with great enthusiasm showing that the majority of parents are concerned about what their children eat.

It appeared that although many parents had difficulty within the home to control the amounts of sweets, crisps and biscuits that their child ate, they were pleased that this was drastically cut within the nursery.

I had three parents who were wary about the ethnic food given to the children. The reason of one of the parents concerned was that her child would not eat hot, spicy food and it would give her the 'runs'.

A reassuring talk about the whole aspect was helpful and she has now accepted, with surprise, I should add, that although she does not like spicy food, her child does.

So many parents only give their children the type of food they like or were brought up with.

The other two parents who were concerned had different reasons, and after initially discussing with them (separately) I discovered the reasons were disguised by their racism.

Although talking through the issues and discussing the reasons fully, I clearly stated the nursery was anti-racist and would not accept any racism within the nursery from parents or staff.

Although one mother maintained her views, she did so privately, accepted our policy and allowed her child to join in the nursery multi-ethnic ideas.

The other parent, who held other very strong views removed his child from the nursery eventually to a nursery school.

Although it was unfortunate, I feel that three out of over 60 parents disagreeing was not a major setback to what was happening at the nursery.

Since the changes, I have noticed how much better the children are eating generally. We are giving them (a) food they like and (b) food they are also eating at home, and although I acknowledge that many of the dishes are popular because they do not have to do a lot of chewing, there are still many dishes in which they do.'

CHAPTER FOUR

Children with Eating Problems

————

— Not hungry, don't want anything! —

What is more upsetting to an adult who has worked hard to provide good food attractively served than to hear these words? There can be few things a child can say that can be more guaranteed to produce instant outrage. 'But you said you *liked* it!' 'But I made it *specially*', 'But you'll be hungry!' are all likely rejoinders.

Adults use many ploys to try and get a reluctant child to 'eat up', including inducing feelings of:

- Guilt ('After all that *work*!')
- Gratitude ('Some poor children would gobble it up'. . .)
- Pity ('Eat it up just for me . . .')
- Defeat ('You'll sit there until you finish it')
- Disgrace ('I'll tell your mummy')
- Ignorance ('You don't know what it is, it's *lovely*')
- And plain old fear ('You have to').

Any of these remarks will probably constitute the final turn-off rather than an enticement. Threats, bribes and blackmail usually fare no better and pile up trouble for the next time.

Meal times can easily become battlegrounds. But there's no point in engaging in this kind of battle. Even if you do succeed in bludgeoning someone into eating any quantity of a food they really don't want (which is unlikely), just consider the possible outcome.

How likely is any person, do you think, suddenly to think 'Eureka! I now realize I *do* like macaroni!/I *do* feel hungry!/I *don't* think it smells funny!/I *don't* think it looks like sick, after all! How kind of Mrs Mustwin to keep shovelling it into my mouth until I realized!'

And yet, it has been known for staff to behave as if the above were a truly possible scenario.

The more likely results are that you'll just make that child unhappy and you'll cause a scene that will upset and perhaps frighten other nearby children. You'll damage your relationship with the child, maybe permanently, and you'll spoil your own day and your own satisfaction in your job. You might make the child sick. You might cause the child to decide to hate that food forever – it is true that there are perfectly intelligent and sensible people who, at age 40 or 50, still refuse *ever* to eat, say, tomatoes or beetroot or whatever, because they were once forced to. They remember vividly the occasion(s) on which they were made to eat the detested item – and by whom.

It is easy to become anxious about a child who eats very little, but if the child looks healthy and is lively and energetic, then it is unlikely there is any cause for concern.

It is also worth pointing out that children's taste-buds are much more efficient than those of adults. So when a child expresses a dislike of something, we might remember just how strong that dislike might be. We might also reflect on how delicious our proffered food actually is. In *Nursery Cooking* Molly Keane says 'I am on the side of that obstinate downwards turn of the mouth at the sight and smell of over-cooked cabbage. Cabbage, crisp as lettuce, is just as easy to produce and always acceptable.'

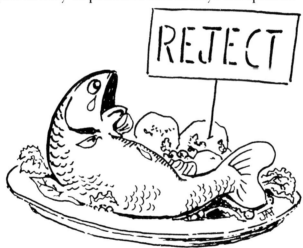

A child may not want to eat for many reasons:
- Genuinely not hungry
- Feeling unwell
- Anxious or upset about something
- On a 'low food' time. Children's appetites don't remain constant – three or four year olds often eat comparatively little
- Genuinely dislikes that particular food, permanently or temporarily
- Has heard something about it that has put him off
- Thinks it looks or smells peculiar
- It isn't like when mummy cooks it – so it seems wrong
- Just too much on the plate
- Food looks too difficult to chew or cut up
- Food is masked or mixed up so it cannot be identified
- The child is new to the nursery and isn't settled in enough to feel like eating there just yet

- Constipation – a constipated child has little appetite
- Food is uncomfortably hot or cold
- Doesn't know what the food is
- Wants to carry on playing
- Is seeking your attention
- Is testing your reaction
- Feels under pressure to eat

— So what's the solution? —

1   First, look for the obvious solution, such as giving a much smaller helping, or putting a sauce or gravy at the side of the food, so the food can all be seen, or cutting up difficult things, or explaining exactly what the food is.

2   Encourage the children to help themselves from serving dishes rather than have someone else decide how much of which things they are expected to eat. More tends to get eaten this way!

3   Be seen to be eating the same food yourself.

4   Establish that dinner time is for *all* – continuing playing or rushing back to play after a couple of hurried mouthfulls is not an option.

One nursery told us:

> If a child says he's not hungry when we're about to get ready for dinner, I always ask him to join us anyway so we can chat, and I *always* say 'You don't have to eat if you don't want to' and I have *never* had a child who didn't join us happily or eat something.

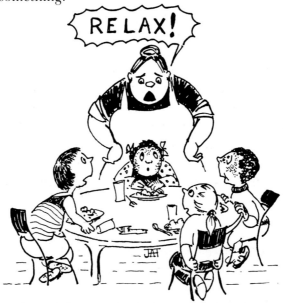

Children should be encouraged to relax at meal times.

5 Do very little else! Really. If a child does not feel hungry, or thinks today's dinner tastes nasty or is feeling anxious about something at home, or is just trying to play you up, the best thing is not to seem to pay too much attention to it. After perhaps a brief question to ascertain if there *is* a simple problem like an overfull plate, asked in a routinely pleasant manner, the food can be left before the child until others on that table are beginning to finish and then it can, without any fuss, be cleared away. Perhaps a glass of milk could be quietly offered if the child has eaten virtually nothing. And that would be the end of the matter. No questioning, no surprise, no anger, no rebuke. NO DRAMA.

No normal child will starve herself. Food is, at its simplest, only fuel – if you've got enough for what you want to do, more is useless and will only be stored as fat. Constantly trying to get children to eat more than they say they want can lead to future obesity by destroying the child's innate sense of feeling full. *Over a period of time*, children will take what they need. By the age of four years, most children are well able to gauge how much they can eat, if they're allowed a little practice.

As to the matter of 'waste' – well, all food goes to waste eventually in one form or another. Is less being wasted if it has been forced through the body of an unwilling child first?

A NOTE ON SPECIAL DIETS

If you are to have a child in the nursery who is diabetic or a coeliac or who must eat any other kind of special diet, it is up to the parents to inform you and give you as much information as possible from their child's doctor. You may wish to ask if there is any such situation when you first meet the parents.

Remember that dietary advice does change from time to time, so it's a good idea to check that your own information is not out of date. Your community dietitian could be of use here.

Most children on special diets are not 'ill', but need what is called a 'therapeutic' diet, without which they would become ill. They can usually be treated just like any other children in all respects except food.

Diabetes

Diabetes mellitus occurs in about one in every 500 children under the age of 16 years, and over 2000 families in England and Wales have a diabetic child under five years old.

Diabetes occurs when the pancreas no longer makes enough, or any, insulin. Insulin is essential for utilizing sugar in the bloodstream. Absence of insulin over a period of time leads to coma and death. Child diabetics will probably have to have regular insulin injections, and there will be dietary restrictions.

Parents of such children may be anxious about it, but even quite young children become quickly accustomed to their dietary needs and can be most sensible and indeed knowledgeable about what they may and may not eat.

The child's hospital will have provided a diet sheet and will have said how much carbohydrate and how many calories can be eaten. There should also be a list of foods, such as the one below, stating how much carbohydrate is in each, probably expressed in terms of units, so that one type or quantity of food may be exchanged for another.

---

10 GRAMS OF CARBOHYDRATE OR 1 UNIT OF CARBOHYDRATE

1 small slice bread (2/3 oz)	1 small banana
2 plain biscuits	1 medium apple
2 wholewheat crackers	10 large grapes
1 small potato (size of an egg)	1 large orange
1 Weetabix or Shredded Wheat	1 medium pear
3 tablespoons of cooked rice	4 tablespoons beans/peas
1/3 pint (200 ml) milk	1/3 pint (200 ml)
1/6 pint (100 ml) freshly-squeezed orange juice	creamed chicken soup.

Diabetic children are no longer totally banned from eating sugar, but still only the minimum should be given to them – perhaps before some strenuous excercise, much as for any child.

Meal times must be regular, and some carbohydrate must be included in every menu. Three snacks a day are also usually essential: mid-morning, mid-afternoon and bed-time. Any unit from the above list would do.

Wholegrains are recommended, and in fact, apart from the quantities of food allowed at each meal, a diabetic low salt, low sugar, fresh food diet is one that we should all be eating.

Coeliac disease

This is caused by a sensitivity to gluten, the protein in wheat, rye, barley and oats. Children who are born with a genetic pre-disposition to developing the coeliac condition will show symptoms, such as diarrhoea and failure to thrive after they have been weaned onto gluten-containing foods. It is potentially a serious malabsorption condition and Coeliacs must totally avoid any foods which contain gluten in any form whatsoever.

This means that ordinary flour, bread, crispbreads, biscuits, pasta, semolina, pastries and pies etc. are completely forbidden. Also forbidden are many other packaged or processed foods such as tinned meat, soup, ice-cream, sausages, sweets and crisps, which may contain small amounts of flour, even if the label does not say so.

This of course presents a problem, but fortunately many specially-manufactured gluten-free foods are available. Some staple items such as flour, bread, plain biscuits and pasta are available on a doctor's prescription to Coeliacs. Approved foods usually carry this symbol:

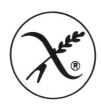

Symbol for food which is suitable for Coeliacs to eat

Apart from these products, there are many naturally gluten-free foodstuffs, for example cornflour, cornflakes, sweetcorn, rice and rice flour, soya and potato flour. Fruits and vegetables, dairy produce, eggs, meat, fish and poultry are also safe as long as they are prepared without flour.

In practice the mother of the coeliac child will probably offer to bring in a packed lunch every day for her child, and Coeliac children are usually very sensible and knowledgeable about what they can eat. But take care that they do not swap their food with other children!

Coeliac symptoms can manifest themselves at any age, although fewer children are diagnosed compared to the numbers diagnosed in the 1960s and 70s. This may be partially due to changes in infant feeding habits, in particular to the later introduction of gluten into the normal infant diet.

Lactose intolerance

Some people cannot digest lactose, the type of sugar found in milk, because they lack a certain enzyme called lactase. Poeple from Africa, Asia and the Middle East are often considered to be especially vulnerable. Sometimes very small quantities of milk can be tolerated, especially if boiled. Larger amounts can cause pain and diarrhoea.

The answer is, of course, to avoid foods containing any kind of milk and some milk products such as cream and yogurt. Food labels should be checked for the presence of 'milk solids', 'whey powder', etc.

In some milk products, including yogurt, fromage frais and most kinds of cheese the manufacturing process destroys some of the lactose, making these foods more digestable.

In practice, the mother of a lactose intolerant child should be able to tell you whether or not her child can eat these foods, and will probably have been given a list of 'safe foods' by the child's dietitian.

Difficulties with chewing and swallowing

Some children may have one or both of these problems, usually because they have some form of cerebral palsy. The liquidizer can come to the rescue here – the whole lunch can go through – meat, pastry, everything. Then everything can be swallowed with the minimum of fuss and difficulty. But do put at least *one* thing, perhaps the carrots, or peas, or some other brightly coloured item through on its own so there is at least one pool of bright colour on the plate and not just the indifferent colour of the whole lunch going through at once. And, of course, the child can taste at least some items on their own, just like everyone else. It's presentation again. Why not a sprig of parsley or kale or a dusting of paprika to pretty things up too? It takes a second – but you have to think of it. It's bad enough to have trouble swallowing – it's worse if you're the only one with dinner that looks like sludge.

Which brings us to the final point about *any* special needs in food: make the differences as unobtrusive as possible. *You* will have to make sure that the food presented is suitable for whoever will eat it. But do it quietly. Don't make a meal out of it.

CHAPTER FIVE

A Few Practicalities

This is the safety-first bit – food hygiene, microwaves, frozen foods, leftovers – all that. It is desperately important if you are not to dish up gastroenteritis or worse along with the main course. There are more reported outbreaks of food poisoning in Britain than ever before.

At the time of going to print, the government is working on new statutory regulations for food handlers, and it is expected that anyone who handles food for the public (such as when caring for children of more than one family) may have to have certain qualifications. But whatever the new regulations say, it should be remembered that each nursery is different, and therefore nursery workers must consult their local authority to find out exactly what the law means for their own particular situation. They must also remember periodically to check that their knowledge is up to date, as legal requirements do change from time to time.

However, the authors are assuming that nursery staff will have had some form of training in food hygiene, so the aim of this chapter is to emphasize a few particular points and to give some information that may not have been included elsewhere

---
BAD BUGS

Bad bugs can cause disease – and how quickly they multiply! In a warm and moist environment they can divide into two every ten minutes, in less than three and a half hours a single bacterium can become a million! Keeping bad bugs out of food is what food hygiene is all about. The chart overleaf shows the most common bugs and the harm they can do.

Not 'cooking right through', not washing and re-washing hands during food preparation tasks, leaving food uncovered and leaving it at warm temperatures for too long are very common causes of food poisoning. Re-heating food can be dangerous: some bad bugs produce poisons in the food which can survive reheating, even though the bugs themselves may be killed. Young children are especially vulnerable.

If you suspect a child in your care has food poisoning, inform the parents immediately, who should then consult a doctor. In the meantime, do not attempt to give any food, though plenty of water or very diluted fruit juice may be given. A child suffering from food poisoning symptoms (most commonly vomiting and diarrhoea) should be isolated from other children without delay, as some food poisoning bacteria can spread from person to person.

WHAT TO LOOK OUT FOR

SALMONELLA

Symptoms: diarrhoea, abdominal pain, fever. Starts 12 to 24 hours after eating. Can last one to seven days.

Typically found in: meat, poultry, eggs, unpasteurized milk, meat pies and pasties, left-over food.

To reduce risk: avoid cross-infection from raw to cooked foods; ensure good personal hygiene; ensure adequate defrosting of meat etc; destroy by heating to 70°C for 15 minutes.

CLOSTRIDIUM

Symptoms: diarrhoea, abdominal pain, no fever. Starts 8 to 22 hours after eating. Lasts 12 to 24 hours.

Typically found in: meat, poultry, meat dishes, left-over food.

To reduce risk: avoid contamination with soil; destroy by heating to 100°C.

BACILLUS CEREUS

Symptoms: nausea, vomiting, stomach cramps, all one to five hours after eating, *or* abdominal pain, diarrhoea, starting 8 to 16 hours after eating. Can last up to 24 hours.

Typically found in: rice, cornflour and meat dishes.

To reduce risk: avoid holding cooked dishes at warm temperatures for long periods; destroy by heating to 100°C.

STAPHYLOCOCCUS

Symptoms: vomiting, stomach cramps. Starting one to six hours after eating. Lasts up to 24 hours.

Typically found in: food that needs handling, sandwiches, cold desserts, unpasteurized milk, custards and creams.

To reduce risk: avoid handling by staff with skin infections or cuts; avoid coughing or sneezing near food; avoid dirty equipment; avoid cross-infection from raw to cooked food; destroy by heating to 70°C for 15 minutes.

CLOSTRIDIUM BOTULINUM

Symptoms: double vision, difficulty swallowing and breathing. Starts 12 to 36 hours after eating. Death in one to eight days, or slow recovery in six to eight months.

Typically found in: canned food that was not sufficiently heated at the time of canning, raw fish.

To reduce risk: avoid damaged or blown cans; avoid keeping vacuum-packed fish or meat in warm temperatures.

LISTERIA

Symptoms: flu-like illness with fever, starting 5 to 30 days after eating. Blood poisoning and meningitis may follow. Can cause miscarriages. Can be fatal in one case out of four, especially in babies, elderly people and people with weakened immune systems.

Typically found in: chilled foods especially those not reheated after chilling (e.g. soft cheeses, meat paté).

To reduce risk: avoid storing chilled foods for long periods; avoid high-risk foods such as soft cheeses and meat patés; ensure chilled meals are properly re-heated; destroy by heating to 75°C.

For more details, see *Food Hygiene, Health and Safety* by A. Stretch and H. Southgate, Pitman, 1991.

— The safe cooking of meat, poultry and eggs —

These foods naturally contain all kinds of organisms, some of which can be poisonous. To be sure that all types of bacteria are killed, here are some good general rules:

- **Eggs** should be cooked until both yolk and white are firm.
- **Chicken** must be cooked right through. Of course, any frozen chickens must be completely thawed (in the refrigerator) before cooking begins. You can refer to page 140 for a good general cooking method. Do remember that a well-browned outside does not necessarily mean that the inside is done.

   When you think the chicken is cooked, do this test: insert a (clean) skewer into the thickest part of the meat, which is the thigh. The juices should run clear – any hint of pinkness, and the meat needs more cooking – and another test.

   Usually, a chicken is well done when the legs feel loose, but always test to make sure.

- **Joints of meat** Aim for very well-done, succulent meat, which is also easy for children to chew. Look at the method on page 140. As with chicken, a browned outside does not mean a properly done inside, so you must test: insert a (clean) skewer right into the thickest part of the joint. If any pink juices appear, then more cooking, followed by another test, is needed. (Also the skewer should slide in and out of the meat easily – if the meat 'grabs' the skewer, the meat will be too hard for the children to eat anyway, and must be cooked more.)
- **Minced beef** such as in burgers or meat-balls, should be cooked right through to the middle.

Pre-packed salads

These tend to be expensive but if you do buy them, remember to re-wash all green salads well before serving. But it is better to make up your own salads.

Cook–chill meals

These have to be very carefully dealt with if they are to be safe, and we recommend that you avoid them.

— The safe cook —

It has to be said that some types of bacteria come from the people who handle food, as a result of poor personal hygiene. So, *anyone* who handles food *must:*

- Ensure that any cuts (or grazes, sores, boils etc.) are well covered with waterproof dressings.
- Always wash their hands (in warm water and soap) immediately before handling food or food equipment.
- Always wash their hands (in warm water and soap) after using the toilet.
- Always wash their hands after touching raw food.
- Report any skin, nose, throat or bowel trouble.
- Never cough or sneeze over food.
- Keep themselves clean and wear clean clothing. Protective clothing must be worn that is kept solely for use with food preparation.
- Never smoke in any room that is used for food. This is illegal anyway.

Everyone who handles food must be constantly aware of the ever-present danger of bacterial infection.

Ordering food

Aim for a fast turnover. A large fridge that will hold all the day's milk as well as all salad items and green vegetables will be a godsend in warm weather. A small-to-medium sized freezer should be enough as you will not, it is hoped, be relying very heavily on frozen food.

Equip the store cupboard with ingredients you know you will use. Be able to justify every item in there. Can you really justify those packets of dessert topping? Then out with 'em! And never order the like again. What you don't have you can't be tempted to use. Read *all* the small print on food labels – you may change your mind about the worth of some things. (See also page 152)

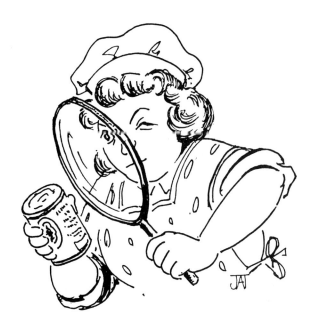

Always read the small print.

Buy spices whole (eg. nutmeg, mace) whenever you can, otherwise buy ground ones in *small* quantities, and keep tightly sealed. Ageing ground spices lose their colour and they smell and taste completely different – and unpleasant! Remember to use all kinds of food within the 'best before' or 'use by' dates.

Having planned your menus, order what you will need and aim to use it fairly soon, so that everything, including such things as flour, oil, dried fruit and nut pastes are not kept very long. Your cupboard may be emptier than previously, but you'll be less likely to 'lose' things at the back and the quick turnover will discourage infestation. 'Spring cleaning' it – at whatever season – will be much quicker!

— The safe kitchen – how to have one —

- Mind the gap! Inspect for cracks or gaps between tiles, sinks and work surfaces and get them filled with the appropriate sealant.
- Use a brush and hot water to clean out the tin opener after using it. Tin openers are often neglected, and can harbour bacteria. Don't forget the wall-mounted one! Similarly, wash out any mixers, graters and other tools, really thoroughly after using.
- Wipe lids of tins before opening.
- Keep knives, boards and tools used for raw food separate from those used for cooked food. Prepare raw food and cooked food in separate areas. Try colour-coding your equipment, say red for raw meat, white for cooked food.
- Endeavour to air-dry after washing up. Any tea-towels should be boiled up every day and allowed to dry completely — or use paper towels.
- Dish cloths should also be boiled, or sterilized in a mild disinfectant at the end of the day and left to dry out.

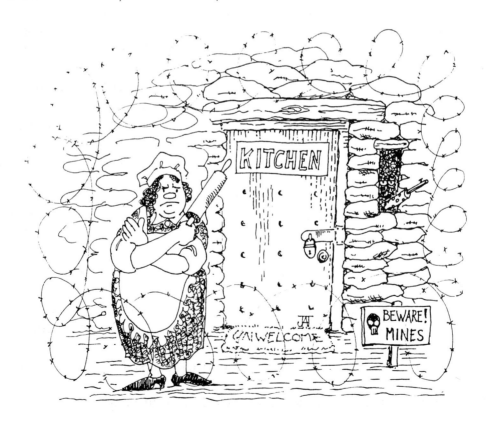

The safe kitchen.

- Don't bring milk bottles in and put straight onto the draining board or work top. They're often wet and quite dirty underneath.
- Scrub both plastic and wooden chopping boards and any wooden spoons immediately after using them and then put to dry. There is nothing wrong with wooden boards and spoons *as such*, but they are risky if they are not looked after properly. They must never be put to soak, or allowed to stay wet for any reason for any length of time, or the water will raise the grain of the wood. Boards with deep scratches or in generally poor condition should be replaced, possibly with plastic ones. *All* types of boards should be completely dry before they are put away.
- Keep flies and insects of all kinds away, also any pets. Flyscreen mesh over windows that open is an excellent idea.
- Keep waste bins covered and empty them *before* the lid won't close. Line with plastic bags. Wash your hands after touching them.

The safe fridge

- Is it cold enough? 1°–5°C (34–41°F) is right (i.e. as low as it will go without actually freezing the food). Keep the door closed! Open it as few times as possible for as few seconds as possible each time. To be sure the fridge is cold enough, test each day with a thermometer.
- Don't warm it up by putting very warm foods in it. Let food cool down first. Cool food quickly by spreading it out in wide shallow trays, covered – but not with anything that will actually touch the food. Gauze pads or the fine nylon mesh 'umbrellas' sold for protecting iced cakes are ideal. Get the food into the fridge as soon as possible, but at any rate within an hour
- Cover or wrap food for hygiene and to prevent 'refrigerator taste'. Use *only* foodwrap or microwave clingfilm to wrap food, but put fatty foods into bowl and cover the bowl with clingfilm, rather than letting the film touch the food.
- Store raw foods at the bottom, so they can't drip onto cooked food, which should be at the top.
- Defrost regularly, as soon as ice builds up on the chiller plates or tubes (unless the fridge is self-defrosting), and wash. Use a little bicarbonate of soda or mild disinfectant.
- Whilst defrosting, check the contents for freshness. Discard anything you're doubtful about.
- Don't overstock your fridge, as this affects its efficiency.

The safe freezer

- Is the temperature low enough — 18°C (0 °F) is maximum.
- Remember manufacturers' recommended times for storing their foods: * one week; **1 month;   *** 3 months.
- Label each item with the date it should be eaten by.
- Don't re-freeze any food which has begun to thaw, unless you cook it completely first.
- If you are using frozen vegetables, cook them straight from the freezer, don't allow them to thaw first.
- Cook frozen meat *only* when it has thawed completely first. Thaw it in the fridge - at the bottom, remember.
- Check the freezer regularly for any long-lost items; better still . . .
- Have a *small* freezer and use more fresh food!

The safe microwave

This is not an essential piece of equipment for a nursery. Not all microwaves are as efficient as they should be, they don't always heat the food to the temperature they are supposed to and can have 'cold spots' where the food would hardly be cooked at all. There are about 800 different models on the market with much variation among them.

Because of the risk of uneven cooking, it is safer to use a conventional oven when cooking food for children. Certainly there are some things you should never use a microwave oven for:

- Don't re-heat food in a microwave.
- Don't use a microwave for cook–chill meals (what are you doing with those meals anyway?).
- Don't use for babies' bottles – the uneven heating could cause burns.
- Never cook eggs in a microwave.

So what can a microwave oven be used for in the nursery? Well, you could cook small quantities of fruit and vegetables – jacket potatoes are very quickly done this way; a small piece of fish on an oiled plate and covered with another plate is a possibility (test for doneness with the point of a knife); and a microwave is useful for thawing frozen bread. Apart from that, we advise sticking to a conventional oven.

If you do use a microwave:

- Keep to the manufacturer's instructions.
- Don't be tempted to miss out, or shorten, the standing times, which are part of the total cooking time.
- Do not serve before the end of the standing time – this can cause burns, as the food can still be heating up.

- Move or stir the food from time to time, especially if your oven has no turntable, to help distribute the heat evenly.
- Wipe the oven out well at the end, not forgetting the roof.
- Make sure the door edges and hinges are clean: food scraps can collect there and interfere with the seal.

Safe leftovers

The safest policy is not to have any leftovers. Try to organize your menus so that you don't have quantities of leftover food. Some foods, if chilled quickly, can be safe if eaten within 24 hours, but you should never re-heat anything, as this is particularly dangerous. Below are some instances of when leftovers can be perfectly safe but *only*, of course, if they are handled correctly and kept refrigerated:

- Save your vegetable cooking water. Use for the following day's vegetables or use to add nutrients and flavour to soups and casseroles. Don't salt the water of course. Best of all, however, try to have virtually no water left at the end of the cooking time, and serve it with the meal.
- Boil up a few well-cleaned outside leaves of cabbage, lettuce, cauliflower, etc. along with potatoes to enrich the stock. Then discard them.
- Refrigerate any leftover cooked potatoes – toss in a little oil and lemon juice and save for potato salad next day.
- Save leftover salad items. Boil up well, liquidize and refrigerate, and you have the beginnings of a soup, or a base for a casserole.
- Any leftover fresh fruit could be stewed and added to tomorrow's yogurt – or cooked and curried: this is wonderful with curried chicken.
- Leftover cooked rice – can be kept in the fridge overnight ready for a rice salad. Don't re-heat rice.
- Any good rice pudding is delicious cold.

— BUT REMEMBER —

! In general, remember to try and avoid having leftovers: they are a common cause of food poisoning.
! Don't re-heat food. Although we may may re-heat food for our own consumption at home, we should not risk doing it in a nursery. This may seem wasteful, but it's better than a bout of food poisoning.
! Food that is saved to be eaten cold the next day (such as potatoes for potato salad) must be cooled quickly, protected from flies, refrigerated within an hour – and not kept longer than 24 hours.
! If in doubt – throw it out.

— The responsibility for safety —

It's *yours*! In the end, it's all up to each individual.

Any adult who is in charge of any food activity is, at that time, in charge of the hygiene. When children are cooking (see Chapter 8), let them see that the basic rules of hygiene – clean aprons, sleeves rolled up, clean work-tops, thorough hand-washing and the clearing up afterwards – are all part of the routine. Let them see that *you* obey the rules too. (Use a mild disinfectant to wipe surfaces of play tables.)

Teach children, too, how one must wipe up spills, especially on the floor, *immediately*, to avoid accidents.

Mention the business of hygiene in conversation with children when it crops up, for example, when protecting food from flies or moving something out of the sun. Regard it as part of the educational process.

Respect the hygiene practices of other cultures. Some cultures have additional hygiene practices, and you may have children in your care who have been brought up to observe these. Nursery staff need to be aware of customs that differ from their own and to respect them.

CHAPTER SIX

Multicultural Provision

This is a huge area, but since food is an important facet of it, and can also be an attractive introduction to multicultural awareness, we have devoted a chapter to some of the issues involved and suggested a few ideas that have been tried and which have worked.

THE NEED

We know that we must provide the best possible environment for all the children in our care. We know we should regard every child as a unique individual with uniquely individual needs; we know the dangers of stereotyping. We know, too, that we should seek to bolster each child's feelings of self-esteem and self-confidence and to ensure that every child feels accepted and valued by both adults and other children at nursery. Observing a child's self-assurance grow is one of the rewarding pleasures of working with children.

Part of children's self-esteem comes from positive feelings about their family and general cultural background, which children need to see recognized and valued. If this doesn't happen, then feelings of estrangement can quickly occur, and the result can be a perplexed and unhappy child.

Food is both part of the nursery environment and an important part of the heritage of any culture. Regularly providing good quality, delicious food from the widest possible range of cuisines is one way of creating an awareness and enjoyment of a variety of cultures. It fosters self-respect and respect for others.

Even if all your children are from one culture, it is still essential to provide a culturally varied diet – not only is it a considerably more interesting way of eating, but it helps guard against feelings of ethnocentrism. Serving food from the same culture day after day undermines the children's respect for other types of food. The 'authority' of the nursery lends weight to what is offered: if this is what the professionals provide then it must be right. Other types of food must be less good. . .

There are benefits for everyone:

- Variety as never before! Instead of meat-and-two-veg-pudding-and-custard as the daily norm, we can eat Chinese, Indian, Thai, African, Middle-Eastern, European, Caribbean . . . and all with official blessing – a wonderful way of celebrating cultural diversity!
- Nutritionally this is all excellent. Traditional foods are usually very healthy; for example, chapatis with dhal, or rice with peas make well-balanced protein dishes containing complex carbohydrates, little fat and an array of nutrients. It is much to be regretted that people in Britain, and elsewhere, are losing touch with their traditional diets. The traditional English diet, for example, of *lean* meat, fresh fish, wholemeal flour, fresh root and green vegetables, herbs, some dairy produce and eggs, fresh and dried fruit and *very* little sugar and salt is a very healthy one. The present national diet with its high fat and sugar levels and ready prepared foods like burgers, hot dogs, fish fingers, french fries, soft drinks and synthetic ice-creams is the result of industrial food technology rather than any authentic tradition. Nurseries can do their bit to bring back real food.
- Food is the easiest introduction to other cultures – a very enjoyable 'way in' to sociology and geography and history.

Also, what a wealth of fascinating information there is here! Britain has rarely functioned in isolation and has always had links with other parts of the world, mostly through trade and empire but also through ideas and language. Of course, the 'British' themselves have always been an amalgam of many other peoples who came, over the centuries, to settle, broadening and enriching the existing language and culture with their own.

It is easy to forget, or be ignorant of, the extent of this. How many people know, for example, that stained glass, carpets and numerals came from Islamic culture, or that the words 'chutney', 'kedgeree' and 'piccalilli', are adaptions of Indian words and dishes, or that the Romans brought rabbits, hyacinths and apples?

One can go on, and it becomes more and more interesting. We can use food to give children some glimpses of the fascination of different cultures.

Characteristics of traditional foods

It is only comparatively recently that we have begun to realize just how healthy traditional and peasant diets are. They tend to employ:

- A preponderence of fresh vegetables of many kinds

- Fresh fish
- Small amounts of red meat
- Unrefined starches and grains
- Plant oils in cooking
- Nuts and seeds
- Quick stir-fry methods of cooking
- Many kinds of beans and lentils

all of which are compatible with healthy eating guidelines.

But traditional diets can be difficult to keep to, since the right foods may be hard to find and because modern foods are heavily promoted. Advertisements for food and confectionary, especially those targetted at children, encourage people to consume more sweet, fatty, salty, processed foods. All children are at risk here.

There is also the problem that traditional ethnic minority foods may not be widely offered at schools and other institutions. This can make children feel their own foods are not approved of in some way. There is often insufficient information about the value – the nutritional value and the social value – of traditional foods, and how they can be integrated into the menu.

It is important that dietitians, nurses, health visitors and other people who are concerned with food in any institution are familiar with the nutritional value of traditional foods and the contribution these can make to a healthy diet. It is also necessary for them to know about dietary customs in order to be able to give useful advice.

—— Nurseries can help ——

People who work with young children are in the vanguard in the task of helping children develop secure cultural identity, and of helping prevent *all* children acquiring prejudices.

Multicultural provision should not be seen as some kind of extra 'subject', to be stuck, here and there, onto the existing routine. Just as you would not consider you had 'done' environmental studies by setting up a single display area and talking about robins in winter time, nor can you consider you have 'done' multicultural provision by holding a few celebratory events and by periodically serving curry.

Surely the task of making every child feel welcome should be part of the very atmosphere of the nursery! It should be an integral part of the organization, the language, the play equipment, the displays, the menus. . . as much a part of its ethos as play.

Multiculturalism is all-embracing. For example, a child with a north of England accent and vocabulary moving to Surrey (or vice versa), could easily be made to feel an outsider, albeit unintentionally. The received message for a minority child can be 'If you don't speak, eat, play and so on like we do, you're *wrong*'. Spoken or unspoken, the message is devastating. Confusion begins; confidence totters.

It can happen so easily, so imperceptibly! We all need to be alert for situations which could make minority children feel estranged, and be ready to step in to counter any unwelcoming remarks swiftly and firmly.

Because nursery workers can have such an influence on their charges' attitudes, they need to look carefully at their own attitudes and predudices – we all have them: and children will pick them up as easily as catching a cold. Often, prejudice can be the result of ignorance, and it can exist in one's attitude to food as much as to any other aspect of an unfamiliar culture. Nurseries need to acknowledge and identify any such prejudicies. They can then use food positively to affirm a sense of cultural identity in all the children.

Besides the food itself, some play activities may need to be looked at. What can you 'cook' in the home corner? Only 'English' food? Try putting in some chopsticks and a wok. . .

Food travels around

- Potatoes, tomatoes, pineapple, turkeys and maize travelled from America to Europe
- Apples were brought to Britain by the Romans
- Rice and sugar came west from Arabia to Southern Europe and then spread worldwide
- Coleslaw went with Dutch immigrants to North America and from there became known in Britain
- Ice cream went from China by way of Arabia to Italy and thence to Britain (and everywhere else)
- The Persians took aubergines and mangoes to Africa
- The Egyptians were the first to cultivate wheat. They and the Chinese were the first to bake bread. The Spanish took wheat to America.
- Rhubarb came from Russia
- All kinds of rice and curry dishes came to Britain from India
- Smatana, sour cream and yogurt came from Eastern Europe (smatana is a delicious sour cream-like substance – nothing to do with Smetana the composer!)
- Cauliflowers came from the Far East
- Middle Eastern spices have travelled the known world for centuries
- And this century has seen all manner of foods introduced into Britain from a multitude of countries.

Who is to say what belongs where?

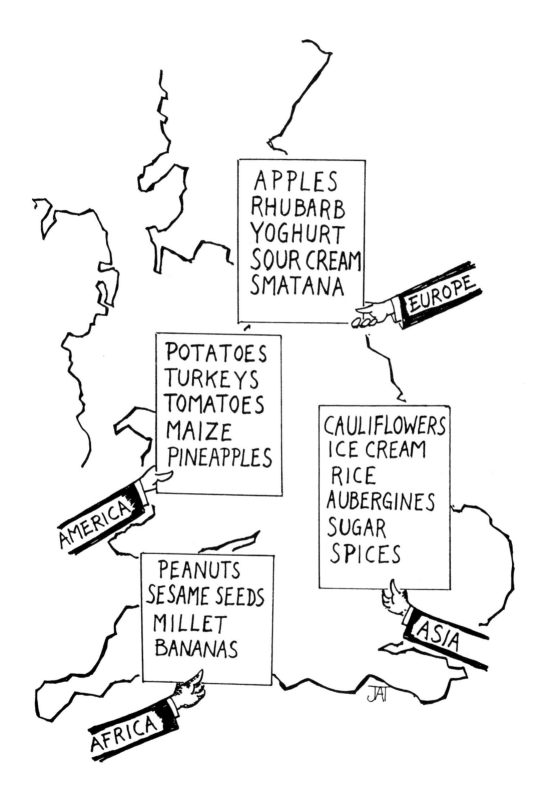

Where some British foods come from.

Visual images are powerful. Are there pictures on the wall and books showing fruits and vegetables that the children eat at home? Do pictures show the realistic lifestyle of different cultures? In short, is everyone's way of living at home recognized and supported at nursery?

Remember, staff can devise their own strategies for good practice. They don't need 'permission' to change their situation in order to comply with local authority guidelines!

— How we serve it, how we eat it —

The way in which food is served and eaten can differ from place to place. In some cultures only the right hand is used to eat with and it is washed with special care before and after each meal. In others chopsticks are used, and sometimes soup is drunk throughout the meal rather than consumed all at once at the beginning. In some cultures mouths must be rinsed out after eating.

But such historic customs, still an integral part of many cultures, may be given little recognition in the nursery and even laughed at. This, of course, is confusing and distressing for the children concerned and can undermine their confidence about the way things are done at home.

— Changing to a multicultural food policy —

In addition to expertise that nursery staff may have, parents can be an invaluable resource here. It is assumed that parents are welcome in the nursery and are already contributing to nursery life. Could they help you:

- With recipes for lunches and snacks? If you do involve the children's families, you might find you have an amazingly wide base of information and this might be your best source of authentic recipes.
- By coming to demonstrate a particular dish or technique to staff or children or perhaps to other interested parents?
- By coming into the nursery one morning to help a group of children to cook something?

This will benefit

- The parents, who will have a chance to gain more insight into the approaches of the nursery and who may be delighted at the idea of coming to show some special skill. They may well appreciate being asked about an activity that bolsters their own cultural identity.

  Don't forget to involve them in forming your new food policies, and do this, preferably, in an informal way. Remember that some families may need translators.

- The children, who will sense their parents' satisfaction and pleasure. Also, of course, most children are absolutely thrilled when their mother or father comes to help with something in the nursery. It will also reinforce positive feelings about their way of doing things at home.
- The staff, who could find liaison with parents crucially important in the sensitive business of changing to a more multicultural programme. Improved relationships may well be a result. Most parents are willing to help with anything that they perceive as really beneficial to their own children's education and well-being. As a resource in an area that you may not know a great deal about they could be invaluable.

— Sample tasting —

A 'taste table' can be a good first introduction (though useful at any time) to new foods. It has been found to be a successful way of offering children (and perhaps their parents too) a chance to try out things they may never have met before. One of the benefits of a taste table is that children can explore and experience different tastes and textures, different fruits and vegetables, and dishes from different cultures without the children feeling under the sort of pressure that could happen at meal times.

A display on the taste table could be of different breads, or cheeses, for example, or it could be more ambitious: foods from the Caribbean or from South East Asia, from Wales or Yorkshire. They can be related foods, such as everything in season at a particular time, or a selection of dips made from tofu. Different staple foods can be compared: plantain, couscous, cassava, wheat, maize meal, rice flour, sorghum, dhal and yams. Overleaf is an example of an ambitious taste table, presented on a special occasion, with the idea of celebrating the diversity of the world's cuisines. The children's families were asked individually to participate, and later written invitations were sent out. The taste table was designed to interest parents as much as children.

Wherever possible, say what the food is and which culture it comes from, so it's a good idea to have some brief, clear labels ready, especially in the appropriate language. In addition, parents – and children – may ask how the dish or fruit is prepared, how it is normally eaten, where to buy it and what the recipe is.

DIETARY CUSTOMS

Food	Jew	Sikh	Muslim	Hindu	Buddhist	7th Day Adventist	Rasta-farian	Roman Catholic	Mormon
Eggs	No blood spots	✓	✓	Some	Some	Most	✓	✓	✓
Milk/Yogurt	Not with meat	✓	Not with rennet	Not with rennet	✓	Most	✓	✓	✓
Cheese	Not with meat	Some	Some	Some	✓	Most	✓	✓	✓
Chicken	Kosher	Some	Halal	Some	X	Some	Some	Some still prefer not to eat meat particularly during Lent	✓
Mutton/lamb	Kosher	✓	Halal	Some	X	Some	Some		✓
Beef	Kosher	X	Halal	X	X	Some	Some		✓
Pork	X	Rarely	X	Rarely	X	X	X		✓
Fish	With scales fins and back-bone	Some	Halal	With fins and scales	Some	Some	✓	✓	✓
Shellfish	X	Some	Halal	Some	X	X	X	✓	✓
Animal fats	Kosher	Some	Some halal	Some	X	X	Some	✓	✓
Alcohol	✓	✓	X	X	X	X	X	✓	X
Cocoa/tea/coffee	✓	✓	✓	✓	No milk	X	✓	✓	X
Nuts	✓	✓	✓	✓	✓	✓	✓	✓	✓
Pulses	✓	✓	✓	✓	✓	✓	✓	✓	✓
Fruit	✓	✓	✓	✓	✓	✓	✓	✓	✓
Vegetables	✓	✓	✓	✓	✓	✓	✓	✓	✓
Fasting (where not specified, fasting is a matter of individual choice)	Yom Kippur		Ramadan						24 hours once monthly

✓ Accepted   X Forbidden
Adapted from *Nutritional Guidelines*, ILEA, 1985.

A TASTE TABLE

Various cheeses including vegetarian and goats cheese
Halva (ground sesame seeds with honey and nuts)
Trail mix and Tropical mix
Bombay mix (spicy)
Bean curd mixed with ginger and soya sauce
Hummus, taramasalata and chilli dips
Raw vegetable sticks for dips
Banana bread
Chilean Christmas bread
Different salamis and sausages including black pudding
Fruits: mango, hunza, Sharon fruit
Onion bhajis
Falafel (made from chick peas)
Fresh and tinned lychees, to compare

— Now to plan the dinner menu! —

The taste table will have helped you spot which foods should be well received and which ones may go down badly. Hopefully it has been fun and involved parents too. But now you must think about feeding children every day.

Aim to introduce new dishes gradually. See which the favourites are and repeat them without overdoing them. Try another kind of taste table to give you further pointers. Remove unpopular dishes quickly. They may work better in weeks to come – or not. Don't rush things and risk spoiling it all!

It is important that your cook knows how to prepare new foods authentically – again parents may be invaluable here.

If you think planning the menus looks complicated, do consult the parents about their preferences and about any dietary laws they wish to observe. Have a range of delicious vegetarian dishes, and beware the practice of having these available only as a choice. Give *all* the children a chance to enjoy these dishes as a regular thing.

Be ready to make successful recipes available to parents, perhaps by posting them on your notice board – and in the appropriate langauge as well as English.

Gradually introduce recipes from all around the world, keeping pace, of course, with the children's preferences. You may be surprised how readily children take to food which some staff may regard as quite strange and 'foreign'. As we have already seen, a great many foods now thought of as

'English' – potatoes, tomatoes, rhubarb – were considered quite 'foreign' once. It isn't the country of origin, but the biochemical make-up of a substance and, of course, familiarity, that makes it acceptable, or not, to the human mouth and stomach.

The chairman of the National Advisory Committee on Nutritional Education (NACNE), Professor Philip James, said 'There is a glorious array of cuisines in the world which are associated with amazingly low risks to health. The message is – enjoy these foods!'

—— FEASTS AND FESTIVALS AROUND THE YEAR ——

Holidays, the main festivals and the main food events of the year in Britain are mostly to do with Christmas and Easter. Christmas pudding and Easter eggs are almost essential features of children's activities. This is fine, and everyone can join in the excitement and fun. But by *not also* doing something for Divali, for example, especially when there are several Hindu or Sikh children in the nursery, can in a subtle way generate an attitude in children that British culture is somehow 'better', and any other is inferior and only of passing interest. What a lost opportunity for a pleasant event, bringing together parents, staff and children with some good food, perhaps a bit of dressing up, artwork, music, dancing and a lot of candles! It may be the only occasion on which the families have had Divali recognized in any way outside their own ethnic community. The nursery, as well as they, can only benefit from such an event. Help to counter ethnocentrism by demonstrating your enjoyment of all cultures.

A good excuse for a party

If there is one thing a child gets excited about, it's a party, and when adults make a special event of some occasion it is a clear signal to the children the occasion is an important and interesting one.

Virtually every day of the year is a feast or a commemoration or a national holiday of one sort or another somewhere in the world. Many of these cultural events are celebrated in Britain and, gradually, they are being recognized in Britain's schools and nurseries.

Everybody learns something

On the next page we give a guide to the religious festivals people observe. We're not suggesting you must do every single one! The mix of children in your nursery will indicate where to put your main emphasis, but do also celebrate occasions and cultures not represented among the children. Be on the look-out, too, for even single representatives of a particular culture.

If you have, for instance, a three-year-old Japanese girl, don't let 15 November go by without at least some small event in recognition of Shichi-go-san. What sort of an event? Ask her mother! Ask her if the nursery could acknowledge the occasion in some appropriate way and what would she suggest? Tackling the matter in this sort of way can bring out genuine warm feeling between people of quite disparate cultures and sometimes produce surprising benefits.

Some festivals and celebrations

New Year, 1 January
Rastafarian New Year, 7 January
Chinese New Year, late January or early February
Tu b'Shevat, Jewish New Year for trees, late January or early February
Setsuban, Japanese bean scattering ceremony, 3 February
Shrove Tuesday/Mardi Gras, 40 days before Easter. **Latin American** and **Caribbean Carnival** in February or March, sometimes linked to Shrove Tuesday
Holi, Hindu spring festival, February or March
Ching Ming, Chinese festival of light, usually March
Naw-Ruz, Baha'i New Year, 21 March
Ploughing festival, Buddhist festival, a week before Wesak
Jamshedi Noruz, Fasli calendar New Year, 21 March
Easter, First Sunday after the first full moon after the vernal equinox, March or April
May Day, the first Monday in May
Wesak, Buddhist festival, first day of full moon in May
Shavout, Jewish feast of Weeks, late May, early June
Obon, Japanese festival, around 15 July
Farvardigan, Shahenshai festival, 10 days before No Ruz
No Ruz, Shahenshai New Year, around the end of August
Rosh Hoshanah, Jewish New Year, usually September
Chung Yang, Chinese kite festival, late September or early October
Dussehra, a 10-day Hindu celebration, usually during October
Divali, Hindu festival of light – the New Year – usually during October or November
Shichi-go-san, Japanese festival for girls of 7, boys of 5 and girls of 3, on 15 November
Ramadan, Muslim month for fasting, it moves earlier each year: early March 1992, late February 1993, mid February 1994, early February 1995, late January 1996 etc.
Id Al Fitr, Muslim festival at the end of Ramadan
Al Hijrah, Muslim New Year, 14 weeks after Id Al Fitr
Ashura, Muslim two-day fast, 10 days after Al Hijrah
Christmas Day, 25 December

Do ask the relevant parents for their suggestions and help early on, especially for a larger event, involving many children. Just ask. If a particular food is required, for example, this might be very easily prepared by people who have had practice, but difficult otherwise. Not all cooks have the skill to cook chapatis over an open flame and the patience needed to draw the intricate symbols of Divali may be beyond the means of hard-pressed nursery staff.

Keep note of what special events are coming up in various families and see if there are ways of sharing some of the occasion and learning about them at the same time.

A FINAL WORD

Don't fall into the trap of *ceasing* to celebrate Christmas, Easter or Guy Fawkes day because you now have a multicultural nursery! That's more anticultural than multicultural. Experience has shown that the removal of the usual party, decorations, tree and general excitement at Christmas pleases no-one and may well produce an unpleasant backlash, sometimes producing bad feeling where there had been none. Such ideas as this represent flawed thinking about what being multicultural means. 'Multi' means 'many'. So let's have *lots* of fun!

If you include all the national days celebrated in various countries around the world, there could be a party virtually every day! See what fits in best with your own local situation.

Dates are sometimes changed when the events are held in Britain, so do check. Remember, there is no substitute for asking around and finding out what is happening locally!

CHAPTER SEVEN

Food is Fun!

Of course the chief focus for food is always going to be meal times. We have already said how important it is for these to be as enjoyable as possible, and we have suggested a few ways of doing this.

One of the things that enables children to feel happy about the food they are offered is if they are already familiar with it – either they have eaten it before, or have at least tasted it or handled it, or played with it, helped to cook it or even grown it.

In this chapter we look at a range of activities for education and for fun involving food. In later chapters we will look at ways of getting children cooking and gardening, and how learning about food is an education in itself

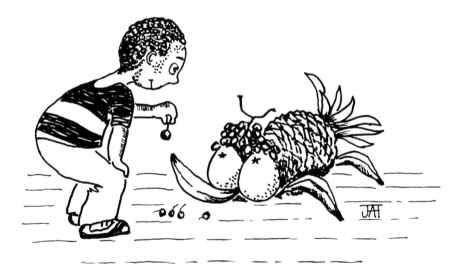

Find ways of familiarizing children with new foods before presenting them at meal times.

— Food pictures —

Children can use a variety of dry goods to make pictures, with or without the use of other collage materials and paint. It's a good chance for children to have a good look at and to touch some possibly unfamiliar foods in their raw state, and it can be a good way of using up any out-of-date foods that the nursery or parents may have.

- Use stiff paper or card (inside of card cut from cereal packets or lids of shoe-boxes are useful sources for small pictures) to take the weight of the heavier items.
- Either make an all-food picture, or use the above items in collages along with wool, corks, fabric pieces, etc.
- Put the glue onto the paper or card, not onto individual lentils, etc!
- Devise ways of keeping the foods separate – separating mixed-up ones is a job no one will want. It may be better for the adult in charge of the activity to put out just small amounts at a time in case of mishap, and replenish as needed.
- Box models may be partially covered with food items too as well as paint if a bit of texture is required.
- Strong glue is required. Diluted with water it can be brushed over a finished, dried picture to give a sheen.
- Give a clay or playdough hedgehog some prickles of macaroni! A black painted egg box 'bucket' will do for a nose.

Perhaps something should be said on the matter of 'waste' here, as some people regard any use of food in art activities as very wasteful. It should be remembered that *all* art materials get 'wasted', in the sense that they have cost time, energy, raw materials and money to produce, and having been used, they are finished with. Even newspapers used for covering box models or for papier maché will not now finish up in the paper bank! In any case, the availability of out-of-date food and the cost of buying fresh will make food pictures a very occasional activity, but a very enjoyable one, and a very good ploy for aquainting children with unfamiliar foods. Better a little food used on the art table than the usual piles of cooked food thrown away after each meal time, sometimes because the children just didn't know what the food was. We *do* waste food, enormous quantities of it, in our society, sometimes as a result of deliberate government or company policy. By comparison, giving a group of children a few pieces of macaroni to make hedgehog prickles can seem downright frugal.

Potato printing

Use halved, small potatoes, carrots, parsnips etc. This can be quite a discipline for young children who sometimes find the careful control required for printing rather an effort, and often want to 'paint' with the potatoes instead of printing with them. However, some children do like it. So here's how:

Mix up some thick paint with a *spot* of glue and pour over a thick pad of folded fabric or thick felt in a large saucer or deep plate. Use plenty of paint so the printing pad lasts quite a while, and avoid thin paint that will both splash and look watery on the paper.

You don't have to cut shapes out of the vegetables – patterns can be made with their natural varied shapes.

Playdough

RECIPE 1

1lb self-raising flour
1lb salt
water to mix

A good modelling dough. Use it for making toy food (fruit scones, buns, pizzas, chapattis, biscuits) for the home corner or nursery 'shop' or 'café'. The dough can be dried out in the oven and painted. Glaze with watered down white glue.

RECIPE 2

2 jugs flour
1 jug salt
about 1 jug water

A dough that children can mix them-selves. A few drops of oil add a bit of pliability and will give a slight sheen.

RECIPE 3

This requires cooking but keeps very well in an airtight container.

2 cups flour
1 cup salt
2 cups water
2 tablespoons oil
2 teaspoons cream of tartar
2 teaspoons powder paint, or a few drops of food colouring

Cook mixture over a medium heat, stirring all the time to prevent sticking. Remove from the heat when the mixture comes away from the sides of the pan. Knead well.

Finger painting

Use a watered down version of Playdough Recipe 2, without the oil. Colour it with paint or with a drop or two of food colouring. Alternatively let the children rub it over the paper as it is and pour on small quantities of no more than three colours per picture, starting with yellow and going onto darker colours.

Papier maché

A quick version which will nevertheless keep quite well: children and adults can tear small sheets of newspaper into tiny pieces. Saturate in water, drain, soak again in water and wallpaper paste. Squeeze and beat to a pulp, squeeze out and shape. Dry finished shapes on thick newspaper somewhere warm.

— The home corner —

Cooking in the home corner is even more fun if there is a wide variety of cooking utensils. Charity shops are a good, cheap source of these, plus all kinds of spoons, knives and forks. Well-chosen and well-cleaned they will equip the 'kitchen' and 'dining' areas realistically.

Reputably unbreakable (!) plastic bowls and dishes are available from the usual catalogues and, brightly coloured, are good for sorting. But do include a wok and chopsticks if you can get them, plus a largish saucepan that looks as though it might hold a one-pot dinner as well as small pans for boiling the peas or milk.

We tend to ignore the actual cooking implements of, for example, Indian or Greek cuisine, even though we may be familiar with the food, so once again, ask your parents! Explain how you would like to make the home corner more 'home-like' for, your Bangladeshi children, for example, and what should you have? You may even be given some superfluous item from their home that could be used – and which would provide a bit of excitement when it arrived – and even more if a pretend cookery demonstration in the home corner comes with it! Everybody will learn something.

'Food' can be baked playdough goods, papier maché vegetables painted and glazed with diluted white glue. Some things are needed for weighing and pouring too - and broad or haricot beans and dried peas are less of a problem when spilled than lots of tiny lentils. Have only one or two varieties at a time since they will probably get mixed up almost immediately and stay that way. Water is probably best left for the water tray.

— The nursery shop —

You need things to sell, things to weigh and toy money in a box. A shop front, shop-keeper's hats, an 'open' and 'closed' sign, and one stating hours of business and price labels complete the scene.

What can the shop sell? Almost anything! You can have a sort of general store as a permanent feature, with other shops from time to time and shops of special interest at special times.

- For example, a dairy shop, with cleaned and sealed milk boxes, yogurt pots, egg boxes with papier maché eggs, butter papers fastened over pats of playdough, is fun and easily set up if harvest time or farms or cows are an interest of the moment. A block of yellow playdough will do for cheese and can be cut and weighed for customers.
- Ask children and parents for empty grocery boxes. The children will enjoy tearing and crumpling up old newspapers (torn into half sheets first by an adult) and stuffing the boxes so they last for a while. Seal the boxes with transparent tape.
- Have at least one pair of balance scales with *large* pans and weights to encourage weighing activities.
- Dried white or broad beans or peas (not kidney beans which are poisonous raw) are useful for weighing, as in the home-corner, but they do tend to get *everywhere* and mixed up, so don't have lots of different things to weigh unless you are content with a permanent mixture of them all, impossible to sort out.
- Greengrocery, made as for the home corner, can be sold.
- Ditto bakery goods.

— The nursery café —

This might grow out of interest in the nursery shop or the 'cooking' in the home corner, or just from a general increasing awareness in the nursery of food.

- A café sign, white aprons for the waiters/waitresses, a table laid with a table-cloth, menu card, paper napkins, plastic 'glasses', flowers (fresh, dried or paper), perhaps a candle (unlit!) in a candlestick will set the scene. The chef of the day (or the moment) could wear an improvised chef's hat.
- 'Food' can be served on paper plates, perhaps brought on a tray.
- At first, perhaps, playdough food could be used, but it can be fun to make it from various scrap materials, painted and varnished and looking quite realistic on the paper plates.
- There can be discussion concerning how to order in a café or restaurant, politeness, table manners, setting a table correctly and so on.
- This can also be a golden opportunity, of course, of bringing in the business of what sort of foods would be 'good' for you to order – and why. The 'good-for-you' aspect may be much more easy to talk about, and to accept, in this context, away from any real food that is meant to be eaten.
- When *real* cooking takes place in the nursery (see Chapter 8) the nursery café could be involved in the distribution of this real food to

any interested customers. One can imagine the cooks wanting other people to try some of their food which they have worked so hard to produce – a view from the other side of the fence!

SPECIAL INTEREST TABLES

A good way of sparking off an interest in a particular kind of food, or indeed of food generally, is just to display it, so that (as has already been mentioned) children can explore it by looking, smelling, perhaps feeling it, and tasting it *if they want to* without any of the pressure that might be felt at mealtimes.

Tying in with interest in other cultures, try a display of food along with clothes, dolls, musical instruments, posters, potted plants and any other artefacts from a particular culture. You may also want to involve songs, possibly on tape, plus stories, or dressing up with help from the parents who have some information. This in turn could lead to preparing and eating some authentic food for fun, or taking the opportunity for introducing an appropriate new recipe into the week's menu.

Other subjects for special interest tables could be:

1 *A dairy table*

A dairy table can be arranged on a green field made of crepe paper with pictures of cows around it. It can include yogurt, cream, buttermilk, smatana, cheese and milk cartons and butter papers, of every kind, plus, on certain days, a tasting session of some of the things, perhaps including home-made yogurt or cheese or butter (see recipes on page 71-73).

2 *A smells table*

Guessing the contents of a series of unlabelled containers just by smelling through a piece of thin cloth tied across the top can be great fun for children and parents alike.

Good items for a smells table

Peanut butter	Freshly chopped onion
Ripe cheese	Curry powder or paste
Whole grain mustard	Powdered ginger
Turmeric	Powdered/crushed cinnamon

This will need some supervision: children may need to be prevented from pulling the cloth tops off the containers, or using them like salt cellars and shaking out the ingredients!

Wait until the end of the session and everyone's had a chance to participate before unveiling.

Tiny bits of such things as the cheese or peanut butter could be given to interested children to see if the taste is like the smell.

3   A herb table

Of course we all put flowers into jars and encourage the children to look and smell, so just do the same with fresh herbs. But this time the children can be taught how to rub their finger and thumb gently on the leaves and then to smell the aromatic oil released on their fingers. (TIP: brown glass beer bottles, especially the wide-necked kinds, make attractive 'vases', and look better than jam jars.)

Parsley may easily be bought, but mint (many different kinds), thyme, lemon thyme, fennel, sage and rosemary are fairly tough plants that could be grown with little (or no) attention in the nursery garden (see 'Children as Gardeners', page 85). They all have pungent smells. *Tiny* bits could be broken off to taste, but beware, the taste is very strong.

Explain how the children may have eaten these herbs before in various things such as mint sauce, sage and onion stuffing, lemon thyme with chicken, fennel in Provençal fish. Such recipes are much more possible when the right herbs are just outside the kitchen door, waiting to be picked!

(If you have some Nepeta (catmint) too, you can say how much cats love it, nibbling it and rolling in it! Not for tasting by people though . . . it's not real mint, only the *cats'* mint. . .)

4   A series of tables

You may like to have a series of tables reflecting different aspects of a particular theme, such as the following:

Leaves we can eat As well as the obvious choice of things like lettuces and spinach, aim also to include a few more unusual vegetables like a red or Chinese cabbage or a Savoy cabbage, chicory, coriander leaves or a few fresh vine leaves, and leaves of herbs too. (Children could be asked to estimate how many leaves the lettuce, or whatever, has. Record their numbers, then count and see.

Stalks we can eat Some plants give both leaves and stalks, such as celery, spinach, parsley, mustard and cress, watercress (keep it under water, it breathes through the leaves) and cabbage. Rhubarb has poisonous leaves, so we must eat only the stalks.

Roots we can eat Potatoes, sweet potatoes, carrots, parsnips, swedes, turnips, beetroot, radishes, white radishes, yams, celeriac, ginger root.

Flowers we can eat Broccoli, calabrese, globe artichokes, cauliflower. Strictly speaking, of course, we eat the flower *buds* of most of the above. The cauliflower is a compressed mass of unformed flower buds.

Seeds we can eat Peas, runner, broad and French beans; lentils of all kinds, chick peas; brazil nuts, chestnuts, walnuts, hazlenuts – in their shells only; poppy seeds; sesame seeds; tomatoes, cucumber, courgettes, bananas – sliced, showing seeds; gooseberries and pomegranates, halved, showing seeds; wheat, rice, rolled oats (squashed seeds!); popcorn (exploded seeds!).

Bulbs we can eat Onions, shallots, garlic, spring onions, leeks, Florence fennel. Contrasting these, perhaps with bulbs we don't eat: daffodil, snowdrop, bluebell, lily, tulip, hyacinth.

Early autumn is a good time to do this particular series, as fresh herbs and vine leaves will still be available, yet winter vegetables such as chicory and celeriac will be in the shops too. Autumn will be the time when you are buying and planting bulbs for the nursery.

And then in winter time you could try:

5 *Food for birds that we eat too*

Wholemeal bread (white doesn't nourish birds any better than it does humans – given a choice, birds will go for the real thing), water (very important), sunflower seeds and other seeds and nuts, apples, leftover cooked rice and potato, cheese, pastry, meat and fat (ask the butcher for a piece of suet) are all good.

Point out that in winter time, birds need fat to keep them warm and stop them dying from cold (birds are very small and burn off fat very quickly), but we're not made like that and its *not* good for us to eat a lot of fat.

Try making a seed ball

Melt some lard and put it into a small bowl with lots of seeds and nuts, breadcrumbs, rolled oats, etc., using about $1/3$ fat to $2/3$ seeds, etc. Trail a long piece of string through the bowl. When the fat has set, use the string, that will now be set in the hard fat, to hang the seed-ball up outdoors for the birds to eat.

In the case of apples, and particularly if you happen to have an imperfect one, impale one on the end of a thick twig or stick, or dangle it from a branch or bird table and notice all the tiny, pointed holes that gradually appear in it, made by the birds' tiny, pointed beaks!

In very cold weather, try putting out a halved, hot jacket potato and watch the sparrows and starlings squabble over it.

6   *What it's like raw, what it's like cooked*

Some children are familiar with potatoes only as chips or mash, and may never even have seen a whole raw potato being prepared and cooked. Many children may not associate at all an uncooked and, perhaps, earthy potato, with what appears on their plate. Display the whole, raw potato next to a little dish of cooked.

This type of raw-and-cooked display can be most educational for children. The less cleaned and tidied up the raw foods are the better. Could any adult, for example, possibly bring in a whole potato plant in a bucket, earth and all, to show the whole potato scene? Or a whole onion with leaves – or even a flower?

June–July is a good time for this display, when fresh peas, broad beans, leafy carrots and new potatoes are being harvested. Runner beans come a bit later – August, September (see also 'Children as Gardeners', page 85).

Some possibilities for displaying whole-and-raw and also cooked foods

Spinach	Carrots with the tops on (spring, summer)
Cabbage	Beetroot with the leaves still on
Potatoes	Peas in pods
Onions	Broad, runner or French beans
Cauliflower	Aubergines

Have a few pea pods for the children to pop open and see the neat rows of fresh peas inside - and maybe a maggot! City children often have no idea that peas grow in pods. Open, too, a large broad or runner bean pod to reveal the beans nestling inside.

7   *A table of what we have grown!*

Read Chapter 9 on how several fruits and vegetables can be rather easily grown in soil or in pots. A display of some of the fruits of the nursery's labours may amaze the parents, not to mention the nursery itself, and may spark off a bit of home gardening too!

These are just a few ideas. Use, adapt, replace and add to them according to your own situation.

Guess the fruit

In this game, the adult hides different kinds of fruit in a bag and asks the children to put in a hand, and just by feeling, to grasp one of the fruits and name it. The child lifts out the fruit and sees if the fruit was what it was said to be.

Find the fruit

Similar to the above, but this time the adult says 'Find a pear' or 'Find an orange'. Again, the child must do this just by feeling and lift out the fruit, to see if the required one was indeed found.
   Variation same thing with vegetables.

The food snake

Ask the children to tell you the names of all the foods they can think of. Accept everything they say that is in fact edible, whether it be spaghetti bolognese or bananas, jotting the names down quickly as they say them. Later copy them out more legibly in a long snake shape. Write in another name every time someone comes up with another one. Count the names on the food snake from time to time. If the snake shape fills up, start a baby one.

What's in the box?

Another guessing game; this time the children have to try and guess the contents of a food product by the picture on the packet. It's surprising how often the wrapper does not give a picture of the actual contents!
   Games about food are fun, but the best fun of all is actually producing something yourself that can be eaten. How can young children prepare food in a nursery? Let's find out!

CHAPTER EIGHT

Children as Cooks

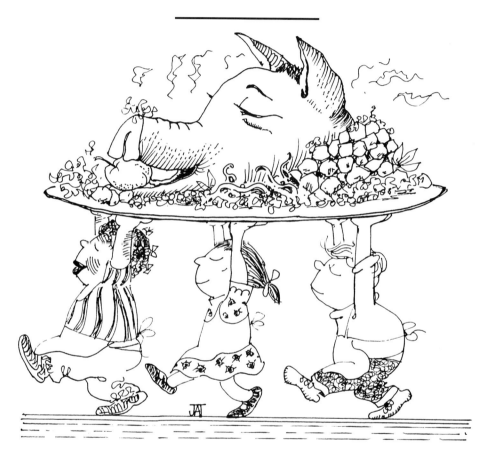

K een adult cooks often say how their interest was sparked off at an early age by 'helping' in the kitchen. Children usually enjoy cooking, and whilst doing so, can get other benefits too: a familiarity with new and perhaps unusual foods, a knowledge of some cooking skills and practice, and also of hygiene, some useful social training, and perhaps the beginning of a lifetime's interest in good food. . . and, of course, sheer fun!

There are all kinds of ways in which they can do it.

- They can cook some item to take home
- They can make something to eat as a by-product of a scientific experiment or project
- They can make a snack for the mid-morning nursery break or tea time
- They can make part of a meal with an adult to help

- They can even regularly make part of the midday meal in conjunction with the nursery cook! This may sound overambitious, but some nurseries are already doing this and report no problems.

In fact, the children quickly develop both skills and speed and become amazingly proficient. Having prepared the food, they naturally want to eat it! Of course this must be well planned with the cook beforehand so it fits in with, or even helps, the kitchen routine.

—— SO WHAT, EXACTLY, CAN THEY MAKE? ——

The easiest thing to start with is something very small and uncomplicated and self-contained – and unlikely to go wrong!

The three following suggestions all fit these requirements and you may find that they tie in nicely with a nursery farm visit or harvest time celebrations, although, of course, they can be done anytime and even over and over if you have the demand!

— HOME MADE YOGURT —

1   Heat *1 packet of sterilized (eg. Long Life) milk* to fairly warm (110–120 °F is ideal), but test with your little finger – the milk should feel fairly hot.

2   Stir *1 teaspoon of any plain yogurt* with a little *cold milk* (taken from the pint) in a wide-mouth vacuum flask.

3   Stir in the heated milk. You can add 2 tablespoons of powdered milk to make it thicker and richer. Seal.

4   Leave absolutely undisturbed for 6 hours. At the end of which time you should have a pint of yogurt for the price of milk!

5   Either eat warm or pour into a plastic container, cover and keep in the fridge, up to 4-5 days, until needed. Less acid-tasting than commercial yogurt. There should be a spoonful for everybody.

For fruit yogurts see page 83.

If the yogurt turns out to be more like sour milk instead of yogurt, then the milk was either too hot or too cold. Explain this to the children and then do it again the next day - you can use the same milk again. The more powdered milk you add, the thicker the yogurt will be.

— HOME MADE BUTTER —

1   Pour the *cream from 2–3 pints of gold top milk* into a screw top glass jar. Screw the lid on *tightly*.

2   'Churn' the cream into butter by shaking the jar well for 20–25 minutes. (Give the children one minute to shake the jar in turns. They can time

themselves on a one-minute sand timer – a good mathematical activity and physically nice and vigorous.)

3 Pour off the resulting buttermilk. The children can taste it if they want to, although it's not exciting, so keep this until after they've enjoyed the butter!

4 There will be a small dab of butter for each dairymaid or dairyman to eat on a piece of cracker or (possibly home-made) bread.

— HOME MADE CHEESE —

1 Leave *1–2 pints of milk* in a warm place for two days to go sour.

2 Notice how the milk has separated into *curds and whey* – and sing Little Miss Muffet! The whey could be tasted but it's not to be recommended.

3 Pour it all through a sterilized, double-thickness muslin cloth suspended over a bowl.

  (One way is to put a small chair upside-down on a table. Tie each corner of the muslin cloth to one leg of the chair. Set the bowl underneath on the upturned seat of the chair. *Or* suspend the cloth from a tap over a bowl to collect the whey. But make sure the tap doesn't drip onto the food!)

4 Leave overnight.

5 Next morning, scrape all the resulting curd cheese out of the muslin into a small bowl, and mash smooth with a fork, and possibly add a *tiny* pinch of salt.

6 Again, there will be a tiny bit of cheese for each worker – on a spoon or on a piece of cracker.

Variation: If you do this a second time, try adding a few snipped chives (from the nursery garden, possibly?) and a tiny squeeze of lemon juice. Or, in summer, it would be wonderful to mash in a little soft fruit – strawberries, ripe peaches etc. — but the first time it should be plain.

— BAKING BREAD —

There is a recipe on page 141, but any recipe for plain bread will do. If there is a current interest in the nursery in farms or harvest, then home made bread can be part of the interest, though bread making is a star event at any time. A few tips:

There are only two real mistakes you can make:

- Having the water too hot, so it kills the yeast (which is a mass of compressed living organisms). It must be tepid only.
- Not adding enough water, so the dough is too stiff and, as a result, won't rise properly, so you finish up with baked bricks instead of baked bread.
  Also, while you may sometimes want to bake a conventional loaf of bread in the usual shape, you'll probably be more likely to make lots of individual buns or rolls, which are much less likely to show imperfections, whatever has happened to them!

1   Dissolve the yeast, fresh or dried, in *tepid* water.

2   Use up to 50% white (unbleached) flour for easier rising. True 100% wholemeal bread is more unpredictable - wait until you're a veteran. Work up to it gradually.

3   If the dough over-rises just thump it back, re-mix, re-shape and let it rise again. This extra rising will not hurt the bread one bit and will be very quick – keep your eye on it.

4   If it doesn't rise much, or at all, assume that the dough was too dry, or that the yeast was stale or that you killed it. So, crumble more fresh yeast into the dough with your fingertips and knead it in, or in the case of dried yeast, just dissolve it in coldish water (play safe) and knead that into the failed dough. Poke deep holes in the dough all over, pour in water and knead this extra water in as evenly as possible. Then re-shape and put to rise again.

5   The raw, unrisen dough should be so soft it's almost tacky. (Too soft a dough isn't a problem, you just mix in more flour.) You should be able to squeeze a handful of dough out between your clenched fingers without effort.

6   If disaster strikes the dough too late in the day to do anything about it, wrap it loosely in a large plastic bag, seal the bag well and refrigerate overnight. Next day, continue where you left off! You'll probably find the dough has risen in the fridge and needs punching back well before shaping. *Great* fun! Allow a little extra baking time because of the cold dough.

Now you have the confidence to begin

First let the yeast bubble in the slightly warm water with just a little treacle or honey so a good 'head' forms. Let the children observe this happening and smell the lovely aroma produced. Don't stir it or a head won't form.

Pour the yeast onto the flour with a pinch of salt in a well-scrubbed plastic washing up bowl and let the children squelch it about until you have some kind of dough. With damp dishcloths at the ready, give each child a lump of it to 'knead'. Actually, wholemeal bread should have little kneading or it can go tough, but ignore that for now and let the 'kneading' continue for as long as it's fun.

(Ideally, for the best bread, the dough should then all go back into the bowl for the preliminary rising, but you can miss this stage out if you're pushed for time.)

The dough can be shaped into

- Rolls (maybe sprinkle with sesame or poppy seeds)
- Buns (add dried fruit or a pinch of mixed spice)
- Snakes/snails: a long roll of dough curled round and round
- Any rounded shape – teddy bears, hedgehogs, mice, funny faces, with currants for eyes and noses and with pinched-out ears
- Gingerbread men – add powdered ginger to the recipe and use currants for buttons and eyes.

Features may disappear in rising and baking, so make sure you know whose roll is whose to avoid drama. Rise all the bread on a greased baking tray. When they are noticeably bigger, pop them immediately into a very hot oven. Little buns should take only 10–15 minutes.

Very new bread is highly indigestible - and may burn the mouth - so wait until the bread is cold before eating.

—— SOMETHING THAT NEEDS TO BE SAID ——

When something has been cooked in the nursery as an activity, for fun, and there is a bit for each child to eat, there will always be one or two children who don't want any. That's fine. They don't have to.

In order to prevent any anxiety building up over the matter, say right at the outset that *if* children want to taste the cheese/butter or whatever, *if* they do – then they can. But not unless they want to.

Really spell it out that it's only for eating by those who say they want some. Say that when you, the adult, ask them if they want to try a bit and they don't want to, they must just say 'No thank-you', and then you will know and give their share to someone else. (Or, depending on what it is, the children can help themselves.)

Also say that, should they taste it and decide they don't like it, they can either give it to someone else who does like it or *put it in the bin.*

Then keep your word. Don't say: 'Are you sure?' Don't say: 'Just try this *little* piece.' Don't say: 'You don't eat much do you?' etc. Because:

1   Pressure to eat puts people off.
2   The idea that you need only have it if you want it removes the pressure. Also, the thought that someone else will be given your fair share if you don't want it, is quite subtly powerful – you may decide to try it after all.
3   Just because it was fun to play with the bread dough or whatever, it shouldn't mean everyone must somehow 'take part' and have to eat the darn stuff. Put it this way – suppose, at the end of a cookery demonstration, the demonstrator came round with all the dishes and made everyone eat a bit of everything. How would you feel? Would you go again?

Food activities are fun. Keep the fun going right to the end.

—— BONES, DINOSAURS AND FISH ——

If there is a nursery interest in any of the above, a demonstration of how to take the backbone out of a fish and then cook the fillets can be an astonishing thing for children, and some adults, to see.

— SCOTTISH HERRING —

This is one of the most delicious fish dishes of all – tangy, juicy, not overly 'fishy' and consequently an excellent introduction to fresh fish.

1   Wash and quickly scrub herring to remove loose scales.

2   With scissors, cut off all the fins close to the flesh.

3   With a sharp knife, cut off the head and the tail, plus about 1/4 inch of the flesh next to the tail.

4   Slit the fish underneath from the head end to the vent. At the sink, pull and rinse out the innards; everything that's loose should be entirely removed. *If* you find a pair of pale pink soft roes, do save them (fry them in butter for a minute and eat on hot toast with lemon juice and parsley. Exquisite! And very nutritious). Rinse the whole fish well and pat dry.

5   *Remove the backbone:* cut through the flesh from the vent down to the tail end with scissors, and turn the fish over onto its stomach, with the backbone sticking up. With your thumbs, gently but firmly press up and down this bone, until you have pressed the fish open and flat onto the table. This will also have pushed most of the flesh off the bone.

6   Peep underneath to see where the flesh is still attached and press a bit more in that area.

7   Turn the herring onto its skin side and carefully ease the whole backbone, with side bones attached, out of the flesh.

8   Cut down between the two fillets to sever them.

9   Carefully remove any stray bones left behind – there will always be a few really big ones at the wide end where you cut off the head.

10   Also feel along both edges of each fillet for the very sharp bony bits which were attached to the fins. These cannot be seen easily, so you must feel for them. Cut round them to remove every scrap. Fear of bones puts many people off eating fish.

This is all very fiddly – but fascinating and educational for children to see. Practice on one at home first! Fishmongers will always de-capitate and clean the fish for you and may well fillet it too if you ask, so you *could* buy the fish and its head and bone separately to show the children, but of course it's not remotely as exciting as seeing it done before your very eyes.

What you *must* do yourself if you intend to serve the herring is to check every fillet for stray bones, fins and the hidden, bony bit of the fins on the *inside* of the fish. (Ignore, of course, the myriad of tiny hair-like bones which are everywhere and harmless. It's the ones attached to the backbone which must be removed.)

11   Sprinkle a few rolled oats onto some clean paper. Press the herring gently into the oats. Turn over, repeat.

12   Melt a little butter and oil in a pan. *Very slowly* cook the herring fillets about seven minutes a side, skin side first, turning once.

13   When the oats are golden brown, the fish is probably done, but test with the point of a knife. Remove to a warmed plate.

To make it into a full meal:

Quickly add an extra knob of butter to the pan, with a good squirt of lemon juice and some chopped parsley, boil up and immediately pour over the fish. Eat at once with creamed potatoes and a little lettuce.

It's actually very easy to do, and though it will be more of a demonstration than a children's activity, the children could help at different stages.

If possible take a few children with you to buy the fish (see also outings on page 123), but otherwise start by letting them feel how very slippery a fish is. Then scrub it quickly to get rid of loose scales and cut off the fins with strong scissors. Have a sink or bowl of cold water close by while you decapitate it, slit the herring open and remove all the innards – explaining, briefly, what they are.

When you press the spine loose, a few children could help here and then, lo and behold, the whole backbone comes out! In a time when many children think fish have fingers, all this is a revelation. Point out that human backbones are like the fish bone, spine and ribs – we can feel them.

The children could help gently to press the oats into the fillets and then the adult can cook it. Perhaps the children could meanwhile chop the parsley or squeeze a bit of lemon juice, or these things could be done in advance. At any rate the adult will have to do the final assembly and then cut the herring into small pieces for everyone who wants a taste.

Herrings are the most nutritious fish you can buy – and they're always the cheapest. High in vitamins A and D and in polyunsaturated fatty acids and omega-3 oils, they are worth acquiring a taste for! This old Scottish method of cooking them is probably the most delicious of any.

Add the bone (boiled up and dried) to any display of bones you may have. This will tie in well with any interest there is in dinosaurs. It may sound gruesome to adults, but children can enjoy handling a variety of bones – measuring a big cow's leg bone (cheaply bought from your butcher) against their own. Books like *Funny Bones* can be displayed too (and read), along with natural history books containing pictures of animal skeletons – it all helps prevent any future fears about 'skeletons'.

Apart from these almost 'special occasion' activities, there are others which could become a routine and done regularly. For example, children could make their own sandwiches, open or conventional, once or twice a week, could chop vegetables or wash the lettuce for soups and salads perhaps in turn to 'help' cook every so often.

TIP
Always stand an (unbreakable) mixing bowl or chopping board on a *damp cloth* to keep it from slipping. It's *much* easier and the the whole thing is less likely to end up on the floor.

— Sandwiches —

Open or conventional, these are easy for children to make. A layer of some kind of fat helps 'glue' the filling onto the bread, but so will other things, so don't automatically think that bread has to be buttered first. Sometimes start with peanut butter, curd cheese or fromage frais instead.

Loaves of bread (use various kinds) should be sliced first and then the children can choose their own fillings and assemble.

SUGGESTED FILLINGS FOR SANDWICHES

Lettuce (washed and torn into pieces by the children)
Curd cheese
Fromage frais
Cottage cheese
Thin slices of Cheddar cheese, or grated (children can grate cheese quite well enough)
Sardines
Pilchards
Grated carrot or thin carrot sticks
Cucumber slices
Tomato slices
Tahini
Peanut butter
Mashed avocado
Sprouted seeds (cress, alfalfa etc)
Apple slices in lemon juice
Sliced/mashed banana
Cold scrambled egg
No-soak dried apricots
Thin onion slices
Radish slices
Raisins
Red pepper sticks
Celery sticks

Most of these fillings will have to be prepared by adults in advance and put out for the children to use.

Eat the face

As a variation of the above, each child can make a face on half of a flattish bun.

Eat the boat

On a rectangular piece of bread or bap, coated with cottage or curd cheese or peanut butter, stand up little carrot or celery sticks for funnels, add other bits and pieces for crew and passengers.

Some recipes lend themselves to group activities. Some of these can produce a good quantity of the finished dish – enough to serve for dinner!

> ## Idea
>
> When it is planned that a certain group of children are the 'chefs' for that day and will make one part of the main meal, perhaps they could wear special white aprons, and even chefs' hats, to emphasize the importance of this prestigious task. (Could a kind parent help with this provision?)
>
> At any rate, they and the adults working with them should wear special aprons that are used *only* for cooking. Everyone should go through a meticulous hand- and table-washing routine.

— Tossing salads —

A lovely activity for outdoors when it won't matter how much mess is made! Two stages:

1 Washing lettuce leaves and other greens in washing up bowls of water. Shake dry (you may lose some) and put in colanders. Tip out onto clean tea towels and roll gently about. Leave. Clear up and dry hands thoroughly.

2 Tear up the leaves and drop into another washing up bowl (optionally) containing a spot of nursery vinaigrette (a squeeze of lemon and *just* enough oil to make the leaves look glossy). Toss thoroughly with the hands so that at least most of the leaves are coated.

Toss in any other salad items that adults have sliced, although some older children will be able to cut pieces of cucumber or celery or whatever to throw in. Eat soon before it goes limp.

Have damp dishcloths ready all the time to prevent wet or vinaigretty fingers going straight to clothes, books etc.

Sharp knives

It sounds risky, doesn't it, to say that children can use sharp knives to cut up vegetables and salads? But nurseries that do routinely let children chop up things for soup report no problems. The knives don't, of course, have to be razor-edged, but sharp enough to cut without having to press too hard. Blunt knives which require much pressure *are* dangerous. Of course activities involving these knives will be well-supervised and the knives brought out and immediately stored away afterwards by an adult. The children can – and should – learn something about kitchen safety.

> When children are cooking, give everyone in the group an opportunity to have a good look at and perhaps taste, feel or smell the individual ingredients *before* they are combined.

— SOUP À LA BONNE FEMME —

One of the very nicest of all home-made soups.
The recipe is on page 128, but really it's only a collection of diced potatoes, leeks and carrots simmered in water with a dab of butter (real this time) and roughly liquidized. A very little creamy milk and parsley are added at the end.

After scrubbing (never peeling or scraping) the potatoes and carrots (an adult should clean the leeks properly), the children can just chop everything into little bits and throw into a soup pan of water.

Add the butter, and one sugar lump – and explain this is the way to eat sugar: in absolutely teeny-weeny quantities mixed in with a lot of other food – and a small pinch of salt and pepper.

The cook can then simmer it until soft and liquidize it.

This is probably the easiest soup for children or adults to make, and one of the cheapest. Just about foolproof.

— MARROW BONE MINESTRONE —

Cook this when the children are into 'bones' (see pages 75–77). The recipe is on page 128. It's a two-day activity.

First catch your bone! Order a whole marrow bone (not just the ends of one) in advance from the local butcher and on the day *before* you want to eat the soup take a few children to collect it. It will be cheap, occasionally given away. It will also be big and heavy – wonderful for weighing if you have scales large enough.

But don't forget to ask the butcher to saw into about 3–4 pieces first. Show the children the pink marrow inside the bone.

Put it into a huge pan, cover it with water, add the salt, vinegar and a bay leaf and leave to simmer three hours, adding the vegetable scraps at the end. Leave to cool. Next day you can all exclaim over the covering layer of thick white fat. Remove it carefully and see *jelly* underneath! And where has the marrow gone?

After that, it's mostly a question of chopping up vegetables and breaking up spaghetti to finish the soup.

This is an exceptionally delicious minestrone, mostly because of the good stock. An excellent main course in itself. Rinse off the bone pieces and save for display. Can the children put the bone back together again? It's a 3-D jigsaw!

— BORTSCH —

You can make bortsch virtually the same way as minestrone, leaving out some of the tomatoes and adding shredded beetroot instead. No spaghetti of course. Stir in yogurt/smatana/fromage frais instead of grated cheese. Equally delicious. Recipe on page 129.

And so on. All kinds of vegetable soups can be used. If they can, incorporate some protein foods – beans, cheese, yogurt, milk, meat. Eaten with a slice of good bread they are completely worthy of being served as the main meal of the day.

> These cooking actitivies will necessarily involve co-operation with the nursery cook. Perhaps she would like to sit in the nursery with the children 'helping' to slice a few vegetables or doing the more difficult things like cleaning the leeks, and then carrying the finished soup pot away to the kitchen for cooking. Or she may be glad of a small break to get on with something else. Co-operation is the key word.

There can be some unexpected spin-offs from the child's interest in food at nursery. Children may take home some of their new-found interests and in so doing may start to change the activities and diets of their families.

In one example of this, a child insisted his mother start getting wholemeal bread, something the family had never eaten before. The boy even insisted he try to make bread at home.

In another example, a child wanted some fresh fruit, satsumas, which her mother had not thought of buying before, instead of the usual pudding.

Another time, a mother was amazed to see her son eating carrots in the soup he'd helped to make – apparently he'd always refused to eat them at home!

It is at times like these that the whole effort seems worthwhile.

Other recipes that could be used for combined activities are:

Vegetable curry (page 133)
Pizza (page 134)
Terrine de fruits (page 149)
Dutch salad (page 131)
The giant's beanstalk stew (page 131)
Greek feta salad (chopped feta cheese, tomatoes, cucumber and spring onions in vinaigrette)
Ratatouille (a stew of onions, aubergine, courgette, peppers, garlic and tomatoes)
Christmas pudding

In the case of cooked dishes, of course there will need to be especially good advance planning with your kitchen staff.

Adults know how satisfying it is to feel that one has achieved something completely on one's own, instead of being just one part of a team effort. It can be a moment of tremendous pleasure for a child to look at some completed food, all ready to eat, and think how she did it *all on her own*. This can also be a good time to cook something to be taken home. But have only a few children doing it at a time.

— Biscuits —

Try, perhaps the Swedish oat biscuits (see below). Almost foolproof. Put out the ingredients for each child in little bowls or yogurt pots on a small tray – one tray of ingredients per child to avoid confusion – and the child can just tip each ingredient into her own mixing bowl (a large margarine tub would do) and amalgamate them all with a spoon.

She can then shape them anyway she likes and put them, labelled, onto the greased baking sheet.

Of course the recipe could easily be done as a combined activity, too.

— SWEDISH OAT BISCUITS —

75 g (3 oz) plain wholewheat flour
75 g (3 oz) rolled oats (not jumbo)
100 g (4 oz) sunflower margarine, ready melted
25–50 g (1–2 oz) sugar

Mix the flour, oats and sugar in a bowl.
Stir in the melted butter.
With the fingers, roll and shape the mixture into little balls, each about the size of a walnut. The mixture will make about 12.
Put onto a greased baking sheet.
Bake at gas mark 5, 375 °F, 190 °C, for about 12–15 minutes, or until a very light golden brown. Eat warm or cold.

— Fruit yogurt —

Being individually responsible for the amount and the appearance of food on the plate often spurs a reluctant child to eat what otherwise might have been rejected. When serving fruit yogurt, try letting the children choose their preferred amount of fruit and stir it in – fun for all children.

You should avoid commercial 'fruit' yogurts because they contain very little fruit (and sometimes none) but have masses of sugar, plus colouring and flavouring matter. If you want to have, for example, pink yogurt because that's what the children are familiar with, a mere quarter of a teaspoon of a good red jam per serving will colour and sweeten the yogurt amazingly well, and the children will enjoy stirring it in and making it all go pale pink.

Having made that move away from the highly sugared (and expensive) so-called fruit yogurts from a food factory, towards *real* fruit yogurt, unsugared, from your own kitchen, you can next start adding chopped or mashed fresh fruit to the bit of jam in the yogurt – and eventually leave out the jam.

Try these fruits in yogurt

Strawberries and a little orange juice to enhance the strawberry flavour

Raspberries and peaches or nectarines

Strawberries and peaches and orange juice (the peaches will take on strawberry colour and flavour)

Bananas, mashed with wheatgerm and a tiny squeeze of lemon

Chopped, stoned cherries (a strong metal cherry-stoner helps a lot)

Oranges with fresh orange juice (and try a pinch of mixed spice)

Satsumas with fresh orange juice

Melon with a pinch of ginger

Chopped dessert apple with raisins (and try with cinnamon and nutmeg)

Chopped pears, chopped banana and orange juice

Chopped soaked (or no-soak) apricots and raisins

Very finely grated carrot, raisins and orange juice

Fresh dates, slivered finely

Rolled oats, soaked in a little lemon juice, and raisins

Blackberries, mashed up with a tiny pinch of mixed spice – even a few will turn the yogurt a brilliant purple. This is a must in summer for the colour alone.

Apples and oranges, chopped

Sweet plums (Switzens or damsons may be too sour)

We don't think the shop-bought yogurt will be missed very much!

TIP

When using raisins, steep them in hot water first for an hour or so. This will clean them, rinse off some of the oil and plump them up, so they'll be (extra) juicy.

TIP

Chop up the orange and satsumas quite finely – it will make them easier to eat and help the juice run into the yogurt.

Gently encourage the children to try yogurt dishes without sugar. These days children have to be actively taught to appreciate the sharp, the sour and the tangy. In traditional Eastern European culture everyone grows up eating yogurt sour, without sugar. So why not here?

— Individual cakes —

There was a time when 'children's cooking' in a nursery meant 'cake making'. It was fun, it gave practice in weighing, mixing, beating and at the end there was a lovely smell and a cake or cakes to take home. There was often fun too in decorating these little cakes with glacé cherries, hundreds and thousands, little sweets and all manner of toothache-producing goodies.

If this has been an activity in your nursery, it may cause some disappointment to abandon it suddenly, so what should you do?

One idea is to continue cake making, but less frequently and only with a very few children. You have more important food skills to put over than cake making. Of course a delicious cake is a great pleasure, but children do not need to be taught to like eating cake. It's a question of what an educational institution should be actually (and actively) *encouraging*.

In addition, you should change the ingredients so as to make any cakes you do make a bit less harmful, but taste the same.

Take a basic cake recipe and

- Use only wholemeal flour
- Cut the sugar by 50% – they really *won't* notice
- Use a good polyunsaturated margarine
- Omit the salt: most margarines are already salted

For decorating the finished, cooled cakes if there's a demand for this:

- Spread curd cheese on the top
- Decorate with dried fruit, curls of orange and lemon rind, satsuma segments, fresh whole fruits in season, e.g. brambles

When children are making their own individual cakes, allow each child:

1 oz (or one rounded tablespoon) wholemeal self-raising flour
1 oz (or one rounded tablespoon) sunflower margarine
$^1/_4$ oz (or a teaspoon) of any sugar
$^1/_2$ an egg, beaten just enough to amalgamate yolk and white
a teaspoon of water to mix

A small bowl, or a large margarine, cottage cheese or fromage frais container
A fork or spoon.

Each child beats her own mixture in her own 'bowl', and should have enough mixture for three cup-cakes. See the recipe section for all details.

CAUTION!
Some recipes for supposedly 'healthy', 'wholefood' or 'natural' desserts may not contain white sugar, but instead use honey or moscavado sugar, concentrated apple juice, fruit spread, or molasses . . . all extremely sweet substitutes that will, each and every one, destroy teeth and put down layers of fat just as seriously. Don't be misled into thinking these recipes are safer than an ordinary white sugar version!

A final reminder on considering each child as an individual with individual likes and dislikes about food.

When dishing up:

- Allow the children to serve themselves as much as possible.
- Don't ever completely mask food with a sauce or gravy. Children like to see what they're getting, or may like the food but not the sauce. Put the sauce *under* the food or at the side of it or hand the sauce separately as a choice.
- If there is yogurt or fromage frais to be stirred into the soup or casserole, let the children stir it in themselves on their own plates – and also allow them to choose not to have any.
- Be fair to everyone. If a child chooses to have, say, her share of strawberries but not the yogurt, well fine, she made her choice. What she may not do, however, is have several extra strawberries as well because she didn't want any yogurt.

Keep food occasions fair and keep the fun for all!

CHAPTER NINE

Children as Gardeners

Gardening is a very grand name for it. We're not suggesting you should drill up your asphalt and dispatch armies of Wellingtoned three- and four-year olds to turn the whole place into an allotment.

But the thrill of making things grow is considerable, and to grow something that you can *eat*, even better. It's also very educational, especially for city children, to observe and take part in the growing of everyday fruits, herbs and vegetables. One might call it the beginning of science education. In general it helps foster the childrens' sense of wonder in the world around them. Growing things does seem to have a touch of magic about it for children – and they love it.

It doesn't have to be difficult. Up to a point, the results don't matter: you're not aiming to win prizes at your local horticultural society's summer fair. It's just another activity, for the benefit of the children, not some kind of gardening test for you. On the other hand, if you happen to have a patch of good soil in a sunny position you just might surprise yourselves!

The idea is to provide the experience of *doing* it and get some kind of edible result. If your peas only grow to 12 inches and produce a grand harvest of three pods, it was still worth it: the children won't know that it wasn't top notch gardening, but they *will* have taken part in the growing process, and seen for themselves how peas come from pods growing on plants – not out of plastic bags in the freezer after all! And how delicious to eat raw – totally different from frozen or tinned ones. (But eat them young, when the pods are just nicely plump, not tight and fat.)

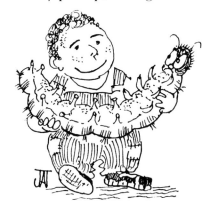

Protein from the garden.

Of course not all nurseries have a patch of earth they can use, but most have space in their outdoor play area for a few sturdy tubs and very few will not have deepish, possibly sunny windowsills, ideal for plants in pots. So there are three areas: indoor, outdoor in the earth, outdoor in tubs.

GARDENING INDOORS

Many of these activities will be familiar already. They are all very straightforward and most can be done at any time of year. 'Mustard-and-cress' is perhaps the number one favourite and unless you let it dry out completely it can hardly fail. Just make it look as attractive as possible.

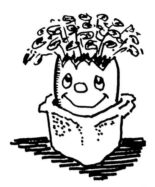

One way is to grow it on cotton wool on sea-shells – cockle-shells are fine, oyster shells will hold a little more, one shell per child. Display the shells in a group and on a piece of folded fabric to stop them wobbling.

Keep the cotton wool permanently damp and water it away from the display area in case of spills. Easy to take home when ready to eat.

Alternatively, try growing larger amounts in any plastic container (margarine, cottage cheese etc.) with a few drainage holes poked in the bottom, specifically for use as a salad item for lunch time. Harvest when about two inches high. The children themselves can snip it off with scissors and use it for garnish or in salads.

You could have a special 'indoor plantation' area, perhaps one particular windowsill, where food is grown regularly for use in school meals, i.e. not to take home and not primarily for decoration, although the area may indeed look most attractive!

'Humpty Dumpty' egg shells are good fun: put a *lot* of cotton wool in an empty egg shell and each child can draw a face on his shell with waterproof inks or pencil. When the seeds sprout, Humpty Dumpty will have a shock of green hair! Stand the shells in egg box 'buckets', cut down neatly. (Another egg shell activity is to make a Humpty Dumpty collage, filling in his poor cracked face with lots of bits of saved egg shells – but this of course has nothing to do with gardening.)

'Islands in the sea' is another idea. This time grow the seeds in a variety of lids from jars or bottles – each child could bring one from home. These become little forested islands in a sea of shiny blue paper, or floating in a little water in a shallow blue tray.

Sprouted tops of parsnip, beetroot, carrot, turnip, swede and celeriac

These can also make 'islands in the sea'. Cut a good thick slice off the leafy end of your root vegetable and put it in a shallow container of water. Keep the cut end wet at all times. Quite sizeable leaves will grow from the top. Notice the colour of the beetroot leaves and the lovely smell of the celeriac.

Alternatively, make a tray-garden with them: fit them fairly close together in a plastic tray and fill the spaces with gravel, sand or little stones or pebbles that the children could perhaps find in the nursery garden and then scrub to reveal their (possibly interesting) colour. Root tops are not for dinner, but they make an attractive winter-time display.

Sprouting seeds to eat

Never use seeds sold for planting which may have been treated with chemicals, only the ones sold as food. Use newly bought seed – older ones may not sprout. Sprouted seeds are a good source of protein and vitamins, and nice and crunchy to eat.

Pick over about two tablespoons of seeds and remove any damaged ones or foreign bodies. Put into a well-washed glass jar. Use an elastic band to fasten a thin, clean piece of cloth over the top of the jar (muslin is ideal).

Pour water into the jar through the cloth to cover the seeds and leave overnight. Next day pour off the water through the cloth. Keep the jar in a coolish dark place. Every day, rinse the seeds twice by pouring water into the jar, gently shaking around and pouring completely off again – every time through the cloth. Leave upside-down for a few minutes after rinsing to drain completely. They shouldn't smell musty, but if they do, rinse more often and make sure you drain them completely. You should have sprouts to eat within a week. Alternatively, grow in opaque containers covered loosely with a lid or saucer in any cool place and rinse through a sieve.

Try alfalfa, chickpeas (also called garbanzo beans or ceci), yellow or green lentils, oats, mung beans, sunflower seeds and organic wheat. Use as a salad item, a sandwich filler or a garnish for soups, casseroles and egg dishes. Or just eat as a taster with fingers.

They are particularly delicious if stir fried in a spot of oil for a couple of minutes and then simmered for about ten more minutes with the addition of a little water under a well-fitting lid.

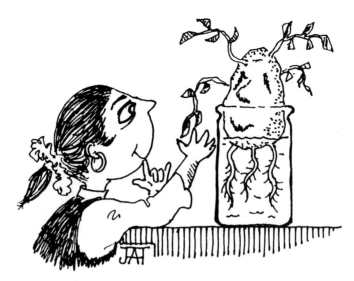

Sprouting shoots and roots

Not all shoots and roots are for eating, but they can be a good biology lesson, comparing the different kinds of roots and shoots that various plants make. Try potatoes, sweet potatoes, onions, avocado seeds, broad and runner beans.

Potatoes, sweet potatoes, onions and avocado seeds can just be balanced inside the rim of a glass jar, with enough water in the jar to almost touch them (it should actually touch the avocado seeds) – the same as growing hyacinth bulbs in jars. Roots will grow down and find the water, each kind quite different, and also quite different formations of leaves will sprout from the top.

NB: Avocado stones may take a while, and it's a good idea to start several in case of failures. After they have split, you can put each seed (carefully) into a plant pot, with soil or compost to almost cover. You can of course start them in soil too.

Keep well-watered. If you cut it back when it's about ten centimetres (six inches) tall you will have a nice bushy plant, otherwise, you can observe how a new tree grows! Keep your 'tree' indoors in the winter and perhaps outdoors in the summer and it may last for many years, become several feet tall, and even begin to grow bark. You should transfer it to larger pots as it grows. But it's unlikely to produce any avocados for dinner.

Broad beans, runner beans

These are exciting to grow in glass jars indoors. They grow quickly, can be watched through the glass, and they are both reliable and predictable; *And* you can get something edible at the end! Here's how:

Soak the beans in water overnight to soften.

Next day, coil a double thickness of thick, absorbent paper (sugar-paper is perfect) round the inside of a fattish glass jar. The paper should stand on the bottom and stop well short of the neck so that the paper touches the glass all the way up. Tip water round the jar to wet the paper, and leave a drop in the bottom to keep the paper wet.

Trap a couple of beans between the paper and the glass, and tip water round the jar each day to keep the paper wet and thus provide the damp atmosphere required. Apart from that, just watch the daily progress of the beans – splitting open, growing the first white root, then more roots, green stems and leaf buds.

Now! You can leave it at that, but alternatively you can:

1 Send the beans home with the children who grew them with information about planting them outdoors.
2 Plant them either in your own large tubs outside or in the ground, and grow beans for eating.
3 Leave them where they are, but in the case of runner beans, stand canes or long twigs in the jars or tape string from the jar to top of the window, so the bean plants can twine round and round. They may grow quite long like this, but will eventually die through lack of proper nourishment.

Or do all three! (See also page 99 on growing them outdoors)

Mystery plants

Try growing seeds from all kinds of food plants and see what you get!

Citrus pips (from oranges, tangerines, grapefruits, lemons etc.) grow into lovely plants. Also have a go with any seeds – apple, pear, dill or fennel, sweet cicely, blackberries, grains of wheat or brown rice, tomato, garlic cloves, parrot seed, wild rose hips, fenugreek or whatever you want to try. Wash them first, and plant them in small pots (polystyrene paper cups with holes pierced in their bases are excellent), *just* covered with soil or compost and keep moist. Cover with pierced cling film (or small pieces of old dry-cleaning bags) to speed things up.

Label each pot with the name of the seed, the child who brought and planted it, and the date it all happened. Waterproof ink or pencil will prevent anguish when the labels get splashed in future waterings.

Alternatively write the crucial information on plastic plant tags, if you can get hold of enough, and insert them by the rim of the pots – and write in pencil.

Parsley

Parsley is a biennial, i.e. you plant it this year and it will last to the end of next year, when it will go to seed and die. Some books recommend this for children to grow. This book doesn't. Parsley takes weeks to germinate, by which time most children will have forgotten all about it, and it's also highly unpredictable – maybe one seed in half a dozen will eventually grow, and then not necessarily very well.

However, it does have the advantage that it will grow in poor soil and, of course, fresh parsley is a very handy thing to have about. You could have a go, either in pots on the window sill, or in the ground, but leave it to adults, who can cope better with delay and disappointment. Follow instructions on the packet.

Remember: Parsley grows sparsely.

Pineapple plants

The leafy tops of pineapples can be grown into large and spectacular plants but the success rate is not high. Choose under-ripe fruit with fresh green leaves and try planting the leafy end, with a couple of inches of fruit attached, in sandy soil, burying the fruit in the soil right up to the leaves. Water the leaves every day – and hope. Say it's *your* pineapple and *you* are growing it with the children just helping, in case of failure. At least you can peel and eat the rest of the fruit!

— Tomatoes —

Perhaps the number one choice and all round star turn. Why?

- They may be grown indoors, outdoors in pots, or in the ground.
- Six instructions virtually guarantee success.
- The production of buds, flowers, tiny green tomatoes and larger red ones is obligingly repeated several different overlapping times in each plant during the season so that the progress can be well observed.
- It's a way of producing a food that all the children will be familiar with.
- The plants are tall, grow conveniently quickly and are useful for measuring activities.
- They make a good display.
- The home-grown flavour is so wonderful and so sweet that even children who don't normally like tomatoes (and this is not uncommon) *may* decide that at least *some* are nice – or may even decide they do like them now after all.
- It's one excellent demonstration of the superior flavour of home grown over shop vegetables.
- The whole process lasts from early spring to late autumn, with a continuous supply of nice events all along the way.
- Parents may want to copy the idea – especially if you can give them some advice on the matter (read on. . .). Getting *parents* interested in

trying some home-produced food when they had perhaps never before considered doing such a thing is a wonderful filip for nursery staff.

- You don't have to start from seed – but you can if you want to – or do it as well, as an experiment. (Start seeds indoors in February, following the instructions on the packet.)

So, after all that, how *do* you grow tomatoes?

It's easy! Buy small bushy tomato plants. Avoid tall skinny ones. Buy 'Gardeners' Delight' (very sweet and utterly delicious), or 'Sweet 100' (the sweetest of all, but with very small fruit). Or try anything your garden centre advises for your situation.

And then:

1   Re-plant into large pots, eight-inch diameter at least. Put bits of broken plant pots or crockery or just a few largish stones at the bottom for drainage. Fill with compost, *not soil*, to two inches below the rim and then scoop out enough compost to put in the plant. Stand the plant pot in a big 'plant saucer' or tray. Water well. Tomatoes are thirsty things. (Alternatively you can plant in the ground in a hole filled with compost. But see the outdoor section.)

2   Put in a 4–5 foot cane near to the plant, but not so near it cuts through its roots. As the plant grows, you *must* tie it at about one foot intervals to the cane with string or garden twine. You don't want your tomatoes lying on the ground (tie the string tightly round the cane but loosely round the plant).

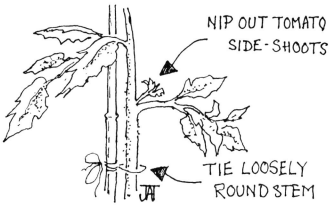

NIP OUT TOMATO SIDE-SHOOTS

TIE LOOSELY ROUND STEM

3   Stand in a sunny place, indoors or outdoors.

4   Keep moist all the time. *Never* let the compost get dry. When you water, pour until water comes out of the bottom into the plant saucer underneath. Then stop. Avoid letting the plants 'stand with their feet in water'.

5   Pinch out side shoots with finger and thumb when they are tiny – or whenever you see one you missed earlier. These are the shoots that keep on trying to grow in the angle between the main stem and the stalks of the leaves. If they're not stopped, they'll grow into big rival stems and the plant won't have any strength left to grow you many tomatoes. Some shoots even have the nerve to come out at ground level. Death to them. But stem juices are toxic, so ADULTS ONLY and WASH YOUR HANDS AFTERWARDS.

6   Every week on a fixed day, after the first baby tomatoes begin to form, water with a good tomato fertilizer. Buy a large container of it, not just a bottle. It's cheaper and you won't keep running out. Water with this until about September. Dilute acording to the instructions on the label.

- Make sure the container has a childproof top. Store where no child can reach it.

This takes a long time to read but you have got a whole six months to do everything! It soon becomes a routine anyway and even if you do forget to feed/water/tie up properly etc., tomatoes are not totally unforgiving and will still give you a fair supply of (still delicious) fruit.

Remember, the aim is to have *some* kind of plants for the children to observe and from which to pick and taste the wonderful fruit, not to win medals.

Cut off the top of the plant either when it's getting too tall for your windowsill or when about four trusses (i.e. sprays) of tomatoes, or flowers, have formed, whichever happens sooner. Conserve the plant's strength.

Poisonous plants

Something should be said about poisonous plants, as some very commonly grown ones, such as delphiniums, foxgloves, laburnum, laurel, yew, English ivy, box, honeysuckle, morning glory, elephant ears, cotoneastor, hydrangeas, mountain ash, dicentra (bleeding heart), lilies-of-the-valley and wisteria have poisonous parts or are poisonous in entirety.

Of course, at some stage children have to learn that they cannot just go up to any plant they like the look of and start eating bits of it, and plant safety, like electricity and road safety is better learned sooner than later. But in a garden specifically planned for children, you must make sure that, whilst using gardening as an excellent way of introducing the topic, you're not putting the children in danger.

We are saying that potatoes and tomatoes are particularly educational plants to grown, and yet, as *all* green parts of both plants are poisonous, you must think where you will put them. Part of the answer here is that children should never be able to wander into the vegetable patch on their own, or you could lose your entire harvest in just a few lively minutes! If you want to grow potatoes or tomatoes in tubs, then position them carefully. A little common sense should obviate any problems. You could ask your local library for books that can tell you about less common plants, but be prepared for conflicting advice.

GARDENING OUTDOORS IN TUBS

If your outdoor space consists entirely of a bit of asphalt enclosed by a high wall, there's not a lot you can do. It may be difficult enough just to find room for the play equipment, let alone a whole lot of tubs. If your nursery is close to busy traffic there's something to be said for *not* growing food for the children to eat – although you could still grow such things as sage or thyme for beauty and for smelling.

However, unless you are very unlucky, you will probably have enough space for two or three decent-sized tubs, which you may be able to get from the usual resources (and see page 95). If you can position these so that they get some sunlight *and* are next to a fence or wall, you can maximize their use by growing some climbing plants that will give a bit of background greenery as well as partly hiding a possibly ugly feature. Sometimes drainpipes can be used to give a plant sturdy support.

A row of two or three rectangular tubs flat against a wall doesn't take up much usable space. Some wire or plastic mesh stretched behind them, perhaps attached to a couple of drain pipes, could give plants support.

If you are surrounded by bricks and concrete, it's important to have as much green foliage around as you can manage. Dark, sunless corners can look much less dismal if some pretty variegated ivies are trailing out of a pot. A Russian vine ('mile a minute') will grow almost anywhere and will cover a multitude of aesthetic sins in no time at all. Early spring bulbs can flower without sunshine, so they should provide a good splash of colour, and so will winter-flowering jasmine, which is also good for camouflage. For summer, candytuft, poppies, honesty, nasturtiums and marigolds are easy and attractive annuals that will usually self-seed. Nasturtium and marigold flowers and young nasturtium leaves can be eaten in salads! Sprays of the silvery seed pods of honesty can make pretty table decorations in winter.

You may want to give priority to these kinds of plants just to soften a bleak-looking playground. After that, perhaps there would be room for a few food plants as well.

Plant the herbs, water them and leave them to grow! Cut them back if they get straggly. All very easy. Children can rub their fingers on the leaves and smell the fragrance.

Fennel, feverfew (for flowers only), dill, sweet rocket, sweet cicely, chervil and lemon balm will grow anywhere and seed themselves. You'll find them coming up in cracks all over the place! On the subject of cracks, you may be able to mix seeds of various plants in a little compost or soil to poke down into tiny crevices, and maybe enlarge a few crevices in selected places. Creeping thyme, for example, is a nice flattish plant that may do well. Don't despise dandelions – children like them, and the young leaves (older ones can be bitter) can be put in salads.

— Tubs and pots —

If you have more space and cleaner air, virtually anything can be grown in a tub that can be grown in the earth. The real difference is that tubs really need watering a lot in summer if it doesn't rain, and you should change the soil in them from year to year.

Some nurseries have turned a small piece of high-walled city playground into a green and quite beautiful 'patio garden', disguising walls with greenery of all kinds and with nasturtiums, jasmine and runner beans, and clematis climbing on top of that, plus a few tubs containing herbs, flowers, tomatoes and strawberries scattered round the perimeter in corners. Once set up, only the annual plants need any real attention!

Use the grape vine

Take cuttings from the woody part of any grape vine in autumn and lay on top of plant pots of earth. Envelop the pots in white plastic bags, and leave outdoors all winter, and hope for at least one new plant in spring! Plant it out in the ground for best results, or a *very* large tub. Keep well watered and train and tie new shoots up along a wall or fence. It is very good for camouflage, and you can make stuffed vine leaves with the vine leaves! Eventually you may have grapes too, if you get enough sun.

GARDENING OUTDOORS IN SOIL

Let's suppose you're starting from scratch. How to begin?

1 Choose (if there is any choice) a patch, patches or a border of earth that gets at least half a day of sun (but see page 99).

2 You can get rid of any weeds by skimming them off with a spade (and composting them in a heap somewhere). Then dig out any big roots and put them in the dustbin.

3 Get a big spade and dig the whole patch all over and as deeply as you can. If you start digging up clay or stones or anything that isn't soil, just chop it about but leave it where it is and don't let it get brought up onto the surface with the real soil. Get rid of any big stones.

4 Dig in some bone meal and peat or any peat substitute.

5 Dig in *old rotted* horse manure but not fresh manure which will harm the soil (so don't go scraping any up off the road thinking you've found gold! It will only be gold after about five months of rotting somewhere). Dig in during spring or autumn.

All this is adult activity. (If you have very difficult ground, could any kind and energetic parents help you on a Saturday morning? It could be fun! Don't forget to provide tea etc.)

In the spring (i.e. April) start planting things with the children.

Potatoes, lettuces, runner beans, spinach, peas and sprouting broccoli are all fairly easy to grow from seed. Don't bother with carrots or onions unless your ground gets the sun all day.

— Secrets of seed sowing —

In order to germinate, seeds need

- Warmth
- Air
- Moisture

Do not sow when the soil is cold and wet. The best time is when the soil is dry on top and damp underneath. Don't walk on the soil when it's wet: your weight will compact the soil too much.

Professional tips:

1 Lightly tread the surface until level and firm

2 Rake off large stones

3 Mix small seeds with a little dry sand to spread them out

4 Depth of sowing depends on the size of the seeds: a general rule is to cover the seeds with soil to twice their depth

5 Sowing in lines makes weeding easier

6 Sow thinly

7 Firm the ground with the back of the rake or press lightly with your foot to conserve moisture

8 Water lightly

9 Keep off the soil when it's wet.

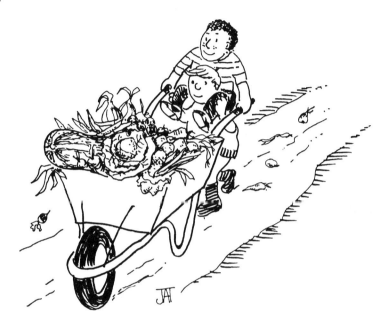

It can be amazing what a nursery garden can produce.

— Plant-by-plant guidelines —

Broccoli Either purple or white sprouting broccoli can be successful. Start off either in the garden, or in some compost in a tray indoors and transplant when the plants are 2–3 inches high. However, there will be no broccoli to pick until *next* spring. It's a biennial.

Cabbages Try Asian ones, like Pak Choy. Plant singly in summer and harvest in autumn for the best flavour.

A Field of Wheat, Oats or Barley Mark out a little square and plant your chosen seeds. Now you have a farm! Watch the plants grow tall and green, then ripen – and you can harvest ears of corn! Find the new grains inside. Grind some in an electric or hand coffee grinder, or a liquidizer, and make a little flour.

Giant Sunflowers These *must* have a place somewhere! Easy and spectacular. Just rub the seeds into the soil.

Lettuce Choose Cos or Cut-bowl which are easy. With Cut-bowl, you can pick off individual leaves and leave the rest of the plant in the ground. Gently rub the seeds into the surface of the soil with your fingers. At the end of the season, let one or two plants run to seed as a demonstration.

Peas Peas are thirsty things, so before you plant them, dig a large hole or trench and line it with plenty of crumpled newspapers and then soak them well. Put back the soil and water again. Plant dried peas in three parallel rows:

Allow three inches between plants in both directions and plant two inches deep. Peas must have something to climb up, so *either* trap the row of plants between two rows of criss-cross sticks or very twiggy twigs, *or*, stretch wire or plastic mesh between strong sticks one side and a row of strong twigs on the other to keep the plants from falling over. Pick the peas when they're just ready and really sweet. Let a few pods go hard and dry on the plant to show the children – the peas inside are just like the ones that were planted! Try mange-tout peas – eat the pods too!

Potatoes Very easy. Bury any potatoes in the soil that have just begin to sprout (or buy 'seed' potatoes and let them grow little chunky sprouts in good daylight). Pile up the soil over them in mounds. As the potato plants grow, keep piling the soil round them to keep the new baby potatoes in the dark. If they catch any light they'll turn green. Green potatoes are poisonous, as are the leaves. Dig up *carefully* after about two months. Use a fork if you have one.

Pumpkins Buy a plant, keep well watered, and grow your own Hallowe'en pumpkin! Also use for spicy pumpkin soup or pie. The dried seeds can be used in art work, or eaten, or grown next season.

Radishes Almost everyone will tell you that children should grow radishes, because they germinate quickly and the children won't have to wait too long before they can pick some. Yes, but don't think they come with some kind of guarantee! If they're planted a fraction too deeply or too close together they won't grow properly, and unless they have plenty of sunshine and water, they'll be hard and woody to eat. They have to grow *quickly* to be juicy and good. But they're worth trying.

Runner beans: Soak the beans overnight to soften (this isn't essential but it is interesting to see how they swell up) then plant each bean two inches deep in a little pot of earth or compost. When – after about two weeks – the seed has sprouted and two sizeable leaves are produced, carefully plant out into little holes in the garden and water well.

- *Remember* beans are thirsty, so first line a trench with newspapers as for peas, above. Then gently put in your plants.
- *Remember* put long canes in before you put the beans in, making a wigwam out of four or more of them, or arrange to train the beans up some other wire or wooden structure.

Watch the plants grow fast, produce pretty red (or sometimes white) flowers, and then beans. Eat the beans when they're about 8–10 inches long. But let a few grow huge and hard and allow to die and turn brown. Open one pod and show the children the big pink beans inside – all ready to plant next year. The children will have seen the whole life-cycle. The nursery now has free runner beans forever!

Spinach Buy seeds called 'spinach beet' or 'perpetual spinach' which survive the winter. Easy. Young new leaves are good raw in salads. Just rub the seeds gently into the soil surface.

Tomatoes See 'Gardening Indoors' on pages 90–92, but for planting in the soil, dig the earth over well first and dig a hole bigger than you need and put compost in. Water it, and then put in the tomato plant and a cane. Cover with soil and press down gently but firmly. Keep well watered.

Shady-place plants If you have *space*, but it's in the shade, plant vegetables which are meant to be grown in the winter or very early spring when there's not much light anyway. But you plant them instead in March–April. For example,

Leeks (for keen gardeners only)
Lettuce: try 'Arctic King'
Parsley: if you want to try parsley (see page 89) try Hamburg
Peas: try Early Onward
Potatoes sold as 'early' potatoes because they grow more quickly
Runner beans
Sprouting broccoli
Spinach beet

Years to come

Apart from the things you want the children to grow every year, aim to have some long-term plants that need little or no attention but that will give you a crop every season. For example:

Asparagus This is really worth it for the foliage, which is wonderful for filling out a few flowers in a vase, and in April you can cut the stalks as they come up through the earth to eat!

Buy (well-wrapped,moist) roots, not seeds. Harvest every spring by cutting off the new shoots below the surface of the soil, when they stand two or three inches above ground. You have to cut every single one that's there. Then, after two weeks, more stalks will have grown and you can cut another crop. Do this every fortnight until June, then stop.

A bay tree will, if left, eventually grow large, but you can clip it to any size. It provides glossy greenery, free, for Christmas time and aromatic leaves for soups and casseroles. Boxes of bay leaves are expensive but, having planted your tree, you will now have the leaves free, forever – and no storage space needed in the kitchen.

Herbs Grow the herbs listed on page 94 where you need something bushy, but try others too – lemon thyme, the curry plant, tarragon, chives, different kinds of mint. Try rocket if you want something very tall and unusual. All good in salads. Chop marjoram into tomato sauce for pizzas.

Raspberries New raspberry canes should be tied up (to anything) each spring and the old brown ones cut down in the autumn. Apart from that, you just let them provide the nursery with lots of free delicious fruit – so expensive to buy. Eat with bread or mashed in yogurt, turning it bright pink. Good mixed with chopped peach in yogurt.

Red Currant Bushes Once planted, they can just be left to provide masses of jewel-like currants for years. So expensive in the shops, but you will have plenty for free! Thornless. They don't need pruning. Pick the sprays of fruit and eat with brown bread, pulling the currants off their stalks with your teeth. Perfect summer snacks. Also good mashed into yogurt or fromage frais.

Thornless loganberries Let them grow against a wall or fence where they can be tied up. Easy. No need to cut back. Use like raspberries.

Thornless blackberries Try 'Oregon,' which is easy and gives lots of fruit. Tie up to a fence or such. Each autumn cut off the briars that bore this year's fruit.

Wild Strawberries will grow almost anywhere and will put out long runners and spread quickly.

There we are. None of this is difficult and can be achieved by interested beginners. It's all very good fun too – especially harvesting!

It's amazing how some nurseries have quite a bit of land, but all grassed or filled up with evergreen bushes. A pity not to use part of the land for something more enjoyable and productive.

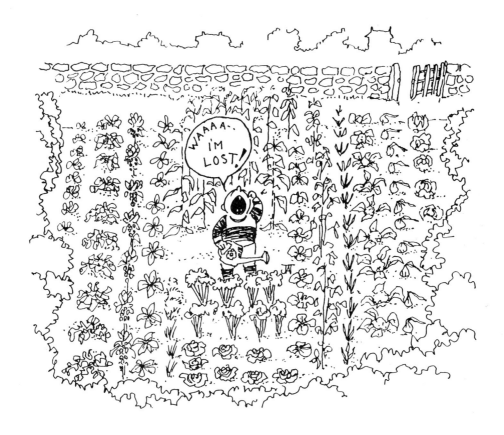

CHAPTER TEN
Food and Basic Skills

LANGUAGE DEVELOPMENT

Children like new words. Children especially like *long* new words. Extending their knowledge of food will automatically extend their vocabulary. Food words are sometimes very graphic or onomatopoeic – liquid, crunch, squash, bubble, snap – and therefore fun too. Encourage the children to talk about what they are doing amongst themselves and with an adult. There are two basic aspects to consider:

Call an aubergine an aubergine

Use the correct name all the time for ingredients, utensils and procedures. Say 'Stir the yeast into the warm milk with a spoon', not 'Mix this and this with this' – while, of course, ascertaining that your meaning is quite clear. It is amazing how quickly children absorb new expressions and words and begin to use them themselves. It's often the adults who then have to remember to use the correct term!

Self-expression

From time to time you can ask the children to describe their reactions to their activities in their own words. What, for example, does the bread dough *feel* like? If a child just says 'nice' or 'funny', ask what *kind* of nice or funny. You may get a string of words, sometimes very descriptive and apt. Try not to suggest words yourself, but to draw words out of their imagination and memory. *All* their answers are valid, by the way, if they are meant seriously, although if someone says the bread dough feels 'hard' when it is obviously extremely soft, you'll probably want to check. Perhaps the child means it's 'hard' to squeeze the bread dough because his fingers are getting tired, and he needs a rest – or that it's 'hard' because she can't reach inside the bowl properly and it needs to be lower! A 'wrong' sounding word may indicate a situation that you need to be aware of. (See also page 107 'The ice hand.')

Of course you will be making use of any opportunities for writing short sentences or single words. 'Open' and 'Closed' signs in the cafe or shop, the children's names on their sprouting seeds, labels in the vegetable patch, the names of the foods on the taste table – all are uncontrived ways of making children aware that writing conveys meaning which is essential in certain situations.

You will also, of course, be using food activities as subjects for home-made books, picture or chart-making as you would with any other interest.

Do remember to make the most of the 'fun' aspect of words: runner beans *run* up their sticks; broad beans are so *broad* (i.e. wide), while most other beans are narrow; 'nasturtiums' sound a bit like 'nasty-urchins' (very hilarious); you need to knead the bread dough; the yeast goes bubble-bubble-bubble-pop! and so on. Don't be surprised if at least one child gets completely besotted with the word 'acidophilus' – the name of the live culture in yogurt. Words *are* fun, to roll your tongue around, to make a pun or a funny rhyme with, to remember and feel knowledgeable about. Make the most of them.

MATHEMATICAL CONCEPTS

You can't do very many food activities *without* mathematics! But you *can* as an adult, take the mathematical aspect so for granted that you miss opportunities for helping the children to develop mathematical concepts.

Children have to *learn* how to use balance scales and weigh accurately, to share out, to compare sizes and shapes, to appreciate the meaning of time and so on. Give them the opportunities. Monitor your vocabulary: just as you would use the correct name for an ingredient, also deliberately use the correct mathematical words to convey exact meaning. For example, rather than always saying 'big' or 'little', be accurate: 'long' or 'short', 'wide' or 'narrow', 'heavy' or 'light'. Consciously work into your conversation words such as: less, more, many, few, fewer, equal, tall, high, same, exactly, almost, weigh, divide, least, most . . .

Describe the shape of cooking utensils accurately. Call a rectangular tin just that, not 'oblong' and certainly not 'square' unless it is actually square. When a word is heard regularly it gets filed away in the memory for later use.

Estimates

Ask the children as a routine to make estimates about weight, area, sequence, matching, grading, capacity, time, length. (Use the word 'esti-mate' as well as the word 'guess'.)

- How many seeds in a sunflower head, or leaves in a lettuce? Make an estimate, then try to count – too many! (But admire the lovely swirly pattern of the sunflower seeds and the arrangement of the lettuce leaves.)

- Or, 'How many of these jugs of water do you think it will take to fill this saucepan up to *here?*' Everyone has a guess – adults too, at the end (very salutary). Then do it and count. This activity will introduce concepts of 'nearly' and 'almost' and 'a little bit'. Don't say 'and a half' unless it *is* a half, or the word 'half' will seem to mean 'anything except a whole one' and set up a problem in later learning. Similarly, 'one jugful, two jugsful. . .' means actually *full* to the same point every time. Checking your estimate must be properly done or the whole point is lost.

Time

Cooking and growing things automatically involves time. You will need to look at the clock when you put your rolls in the oven and work out when to take them out. Discuss this with the children so they become accustomed to hearing words like 'minutes', 'o'clock,' 'half past,' and learn that clocks have faces and hands!

Time short jobs, like one minute per child to shake the jar to churn the butter, with a one minute sand-timer. How many days did it take the seeds to sprout, the beans to run up the canes, the potatoes to come up? How long did it take to make the fruit buns from start to finish – and how long to eat them? (Goodness!)

Just for fun, 'tell the time' with dandelion clocks, which children still enjoy doing.

Weighing

Sometimes you will need to weigh exact amounts for particular recipes and want to use weights.

You can also use the scales to check on estimates. If the recipe says '5 medium potatoes, 4 large carrots and 2 leeks', ask the children which of those will be the heaviest, which the lightest, and then weigh one against the other to find out. Weigh without scales! Show the children how to hold a potato in either hand, to see which is the heavier.

Measuring

Opportunities for measuring will arise continually when you start growing things, you just have to remember to make the most of them! If you have six avocado plants at different heights, you could invite the children's suggestions of how to put them in a line in order of height and talk about 'tallest', 'shortest' and so on. You could measure them with bricks or whatever or get a tape measure or rule and see how many centimetres the tallest and shortest ones are, if there is sufficient interest.

Perhaps keep a weekly record of how tall your new plants are. Really tall things like the runner beans (even those grown indoors, thin but tall,) or giant sunflowers are of course amazing. Just think – you start off with a seed you can hold in your hand, and soon the seed has grown into something as tall as *you* . . . and then even taller! (Pull them up at the end of the season, lay them on the floor and see how many children can fit along them sitting down, lying end to end . . .)

Sorting

Use opportunities for sorting ingredients into groups or 'sets' of the same kind of item. If you are making mixed vegetable soup, put the courgettes, carrots, onions, leeks and parsley in a bag, and have the children sort them into sets. Some sets will be bigger than others, of course. If you sort the vegetables out yourself for the children to scrub and chop up, you have lost an opportunity. Or, the ingredients that need chopping can all go into one bowl, and things that will be cooked whole (perhaps some very small potatoes or baby carrots or fresh peas) into another.

Symmetry

When preparing fruits and vegetables, sometimes make a point of cutting an apple, pear, tomato, cauliflower or red pepper, etc., in half and noticing the *symmetry*, that the two halves are *symmetrical*. Use the words. Repeat them often.

One-to-one correspondence

This crops up all the time – you just have to make sure you make the most of it and arrange to have situations in which you foster understanding of this concept.

If the children help to lay the tables for dinner, they will soon be able to put a spoon by every chair, a beaker by every spoon, a plate of bread for each table. Also, when cooking, everyone in the group will need one mixing bowl, one damp cloth to go underneath it, one spoon etc.

Of course, getting children to help in this way teaches a measure of independence, as well as (after you have taken the time to set it up) some genuine help for the hard-working staff.

Of course, food activities will involve ordinary counting. But as well as one-two-three, don't forget to use opportunities for ordinal numbers, first-second-third, instead whenever suitable. These sometimes get neglected.

Science is really all about 'What happens if . . .?' and 'Why does so-and-so happen?' It's about being curious. It should be fascinating. It should be fun to try and find out something and we should try at all costs to preserve this sense of fun and the child's sense of wonder. The 'success' of an experiment in adult terms is less important at this stage than the enjoyment of doing it.

The whole business of food, cooking it and growing it, is rather like a scientific experiment. Food and plants behave according to scientific principles. One needn't get too involved in theory, but there are various little 'experiments' that young children can do in conjunction with preparing a dish.

Absorbency

- Soak beans overnight in cold water ready for growing. Next day compare them with unsoaked beans. Why are the soaked ones so much bigger?
- Sprinkle bran or rolled oats into a dish. Just cover with water. Inspect after 10 minutes. Compare with unsoaked. What has happened? Where is the water?
- When growing beans in jars, notice how the absorbent paper round the sides soaks up the water – and changes colour as it does so. Do things always get darker when they get wet?
- Where does the water go when making vegetables out of papier maché?
- Soak raisins in hot water before adding to recipes. Notice how plump the raisins become after an hour or so. Why?
- Why are hard little grains of rice so soft after being cooked? Soak dry bread in water. What happens to it?
- Sprinkle powdered gelatine onto a little cold water. What a difference! Why?

Remember to keep back a few un-soaked samples for comparison.

Solubility

- Stir sugar and salt into separate containers of warm water. They disappear! Or are they still there? Taste and see, along with plain warm water. So what has happened?
- Soak gelatine in cold water as above, then heat very gently to dissolve completely. Let the children smell it, too. What does it smell like? Stir it into orange juice and make a jelly! And later, of course, eat it. Make sure the children have a chance to see the gradual setting process.

- Dissolve powdered milk, cocoa, coffee granules in cold water, separately. Heat altogether and drink.
- Crumble a stock cube into water and stir in. Heat (and taste).
- Compare dissolving various items mentioned above in both hot and cold water. Which dissolves them more thoroughly?
- Try to dissolve an apple, a banana, a potato. What happens? Why?

Evaporation

- Where does the water go when you boil potatoes?
- Boil some water on its own in a small saucepan until it has all gone – but where?

(NB Children should not go into the nursery kitchen while any cooking or food preparation is being done. Even so, you may prefer to do this experiment on your own in the kitchen and just bring back the pan to show the children, or let them wipe their finger tips on the white residue on the (cooled) pan. What is *that*? Taste it. (Or try evaporating water in the sun.)

Mixing oil and water

- Pour oil and water into a screw top, lidded jar. Watch them separate. Shake and see if they separate again. Can anyone make them stay mixed?
- Repeat with creamy milk – although the waiting times are longer. Shake up and drink.
- Repeat with oil and a little lemon juice. Add a little seasoning (optionally) and use to dress a salad.

Oxidation

- Cut some slices of apple or banana or scrape a carrot. Wait about half an hour. What happens?
- Repeat the above experiment but toss the food in lemon juice immediately after cutting. What happens now?
- Repeat using water or oil. What happens?

Finally, eat the fruit and the carrot. (You could remove the discoloured, oxidized parts, but they're quite safe to eat – just less nutritious!)

Freezing and melting

The Ice Hand Pour water into a rubber glove to about $7/8$ full, tie up round the wrist and freeze overnight. Next day, let the children watch as you *carefully* peel off the glove to reveal an ice hand. Everyone can 'shake hands' with it and watch it gradually melt and lose its fingers.

This is also a wonderful opportunity for language develpment:

Pass either the hand or any sizeable piece of ice round a group of children. Each child has to say what it feels like – *while he or she is holding it* – and then quickly pass it on. *All* words are valid, including the word 'hot' which you may well hear. If you can, jot down the words as the children say them and read the list back to them. An enjoyable activity, especially in seasonal weather.

Variation: Scrub out the glove, then repeat the experiment with fruit juice. Lollipop fingers to suck!

The effect of sunlight on plants

- Sprout some turnip tops or potatoes, some in good light, some in poor light and some in a dark cupboard. Compare them after they've grown. Bring the cupboard plants into the light and see what gradually happens.
- Sprout a whole carrot wrapped in damp paper inside a plastic bag (keep it in a cold place). After a week or two, long white roots will grow. Then bring into the light and observe what happens.

—— Do plants know where daylight is? ——

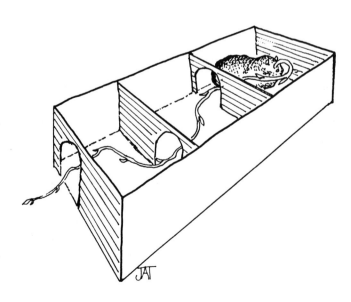

The potato maze.

- *Make a potato maze:* take a small shoe box with a lid. Cut two pieces of card the same size as the end of the box. Cut an archway in each, but in different places and fix across the shoe box with sticky tape. Make a hole about one inch square at one end of the box. Put the potato in the box at the end that does not have the hole in it. Put on the lid and seal. Leave undisturbed until you see potato sprouts poking out of the hole in the box! This will take several weeks. Remove the lid to see how the potato worked out the way to the light.
- Notice if any plants you have grown lean towards the window. What happens if you turn these plants round?

Do plants need water?

- Take two similar ready-sprouted vegetable tops, or two small bunches of parsley. Stand them next to each other, one in water, one not. What happens? Can you revive the drooping plant. How?

Do plants know which way is up?

- Fill a glass jar with cotton wool and fill with water. Drain. Press two or three beans between the cotton wool and the jar, so that they are about half way down the jar. Watch them sprout – roots down and shoots up. Then turn the jar upside-down and wait a few days. Keep the cotton wool moist. What happens to the direction of the roots and shoots? Do these little plants know which way is up?

— Can you make water go up – and stay up? —

- Plants can! Right up to their topmost leaves. One morning, colour some water in a jar with a few drops of ink or food colouring. Into it put a stalk of celery, newly cut. Later in the day see what has happened. Cut the celery stalk into two or three pieces and see how the water travelled up to the leaves.
- Can *you* make water go up and stay there? Yes! You can suck it up through a straw. Fasten two straws together end to end with masking tape and see if you can suck it up through the length of two straws. Then try three, four . . . How many straws fastened together in a line can you suck up the water through? (Surround this activity with plenty of newspapers . . .)

— Do nuts really contain oil? —

- A very vigorous and noisy activity, maybe best done out of doors.

Blanch some almonds. (Soak in hot water for several minutes. Remove, cool and squirt each almond out of its skin. Try not to lose too many.)

Put the blanched almonds inside a heavy-duty plastic bag. Beat and roll with a rolling pin. Keep shaking the bag so all the almonds get a fair beating.

When no-one has any energy left to carry on, remove the mass of pounded nuts and see how sticky and oily they are – almond butter! Eat on bread or with fingers just as it is.

- Try with peanuts if you can get them without skins. (The ones you buy may be too dry, but that is essentially how peanut butter is made.)

NB Young children can choke on nuts, so make sure no tasting takes place before the nuts are pounded well into nut butter.

— Soup that falls down —

Do this experiment when you are making a vegetable soup such as Soup à la Bonne Femme (page 128) or Greek Lentil Soup (page 128). Take some of the Soup à la Bonne Femme for this experiment *before* it has been liquidized.

- Put the soup into a glass jar. Leave undisturbed for a few hours. The small particles in the food will slowly fall down to the bottom of the jar and the water will be clearly visible on top. Why did it take them so long to fall down? (Also try with stewed apples.)

Let the children force the food through a sieve over a bowl, pushing through with the end of a rolling pin, to make a puree. What happens when you leave a puree to stand a few hours? Why? Eat the puree.

—————— MUSIC, DANCE AND DRAMA ——————

A frequent combination activity with young children, music, dance and drama are often at their most enjoyable when they arise spontaneously.

Music

One of the nice things about cooking is that you can sing while you do it. Any well-liked song that you or the children want to spontaneously burst into will do, but you can also make up appropriate words to fit some easy tune. For example,

> This is the way we knead the dough
> > kneaded the dough
> > kneaded the dough

to the tune of 'Here We Go Round The Mulberry Bush'.

Make up more verses, encouraging children's suggestions, such as:

> 'This is the way the bread will rise
> > – we'll punch it down
> > – we'll eat the bread.

Sing the whole song later too, with an appropriate mime.

Or: Browny bread is good for you
Or: Browny bread is yum-yum-yum

to the tune of 'London Bridge Is Falling Down'.

These other well-known tunes are useful for singing your own newly composed words to:

Twinkle Twinkle Little Star	The Train Is A-Coming
There Were Ten In The Bed	Aiken Drum
In And Out The Dusky Bluebells	One Finger One Thumb Keep Moving
Skip To My Lou	This Old Man

Improvise traditional folk instruments by filling lidded containers with such things as rice, large beans, small beans, lentils, tea and salt for use as shakers. Let the children help. Cover the containers with washable stick-on fabric or with gloss paint. Have a 'Listen to the food' corner!

Dance and drama

This is mostly a play activity at the nursery stage, but adults can make suggestions that will encourage self-expression and imagination in this area. After doing an activity – act it! 'Let's Pretend' is fun.

- So, after watching yeast fizzing away, the children may readily respond to a suggestion that they pretend they're the yeast, fizzing and popping. If you can improvise something simple on the piano or can quickly fish out a record or tape (perhaps planned for in advance?), a spontaneous 'yeast-dance' might take place.

  You can then follow that up with another appropriate dance, or a song, or a finger play, or a story connected with the bread-making activity – or not, depending on the level of interest. A dramatic activity that lasts a few seconds can be just enough.

- You could act a short, simple story with the children, with or without music. For example,

Skipping to the shop to buy food, swinging a shopping basket
Acting putting the food into the basket and paying
Walking home with the very heavy basket
Putting down the basket
Dancing round the basket
Now tired, sitting down

— Songs, rhymes and finger plays involving food —

Little Miss Muffet
Little Jack Horner
Simple Simon
The Queen of Hearts
Sing a Song of Sixpence
Jack Sprat
Oranges and lemons
One Potato, Two Potato
Pat-a-Cake
Five Rosy Apples by the Cottage Door
Mix a Pancake, stir a Pancake
A Browny Egg for Easter
Old Mother Hubbard
There was an Old Woman who Swallowed a Fly

May we suggest it is now time to drop:-
Five current buns in the baker's shop
Big and round with sugar on top?

How about:

Humpty Dumpty sat on the wall
Humpty Dumpty had a great fall
All the king's horses
And all the king's men
Said 'Scrambled eggs
For dinner again!

There was a young man of St Just
Who ate apple pie till he bust;
It wasn't the fru-it
That caused him to do it,
What finished him off was the crust

A gentleman dining at Crewe
Found a rather large mouse in his stew;
Said the waiter 'Don't shout
'And wave it about
'Or the rest will be wanting one too'

There was an old person whose habits
Induced him to feed upon rabbits
When he'd eaten eighteen
He turned perfectly green
Upon which he relinquished those habits.

There was a little seed
It was very small indeed
But it made a little plant
And it grew, grew, grew;

The plant became a vine
It had blossoms eighty-nine;
While this tale is very strange
It is true, true, true!

This last one comes from *The Magic Of Music, Book 1*, Ginn & Co., Home Office, Boston, Mass 02117, USA. The book has a good selection of simple and delightful songs for young children.

Old Mister Rabbit
You've got a mighty habit
Of jumping in the garden
And eating all my cabbage

My horses aren't hungry
They won't eat your hay
So I'll get on my pony
I'm going away

Old Aunt Kate
She bake a cake
She bake it 'hind the garden gate
She sift the meal
She gimme the dust
She bake the bread
She gimme the crust
She eat the meat
She gimme the skin
And that's the way she took me in

The music for these last three can be found in *American Folk Songs For Children* by Ruth Crawford Seeger, Doubleday & Co, New York.

Build a house of sandwiches
Thick and thin,
Make a little chimney
Of tomato skin
Lettuce for the windows,
Pancakes for the floor,
Let's walk in
Through the big banana door!

— Stories involving food —

Dick Bruna	The Apple	Methuen
John Burningham	Avocado Baby	Picture Lions
	The Baked Bean Queen	Picture Lions
Eric Carle	The Very Hungry Caterpillar	Picture Puffins
Paul Dowling	Beans on Toast	Picture Lions
	Eggs	Picture Lions
	Hot Dog	Picture Lions
Audrey Fletcher	Abrar's Holiday	Cambridge University Press
Sarah Garland	Having a Picnic	Picture Puffins
Helme Heine	The Most Beautiful Egg In The World	Picture Lions
Pat Hutchins	Don't Forget the Bacon	Picture Puffins
S. Jenkin-Pearce	Bad Boris and the Birthday	Arrow Books
Keiko Kasza	The Wolf's Chicken Stew	Mammoth
Thelma Lambert	Benny the Boaster	Hamish Hamilton Cartwheel Series
Margaret Mahy	The Witch in the Cherry Tree*	Picture Puffins
	Jam	Mammoth
David McKee	King Rollo and the Dishes	Beaver Books
	King Rollo and the Breakfast	Beaver Books
Frances Mesley	The Dinosaur's Eggs	Harper & Row
Jane Miller	Farm Alphabet Book	Picturemac
Nicoll & Pienkowski	Meg's Eggs	Picture Puffins
Susan Heyboer O'Keefe	One Hungry Monster	Little Brown & Co
David Pelham	Sam's Sandwich	Jonathon Cape
Jan Pienkowski	Food	Heinemann
Beatrix Potter	The Tale of Peter Rabbit	Warne & Co.
	The Tale of Squirrel Nutkin	Warne & Co.
Maurice Sendak	Chicken Soup With Rice	Harper and Row (Nutshell Library)
Dr Seuss	Green Eggs and Ham	Collins
	One Fish, Two Fish, Red Fish, Blue Fish	Collins
Brian Wildsmith	The Apple Bird	Oxford University Press
Cindy Wheeler	Marmalade's Picnic	Picture Corgis

*The book contains a reliable and easy recipe for gingerbread men, suitable for children to make.

Traditional Stories

The Little Red Hen
The Magic Porridge Pot
Jack And The Beanstalk
The Three Bears
The Enormous Turnip
The Gingerbread Man
The Runaway Pancake
Stone Soup
The Three Wishes/Magic Sausage
Chicken Licken

Also aim to have a selection of well-illustrated factual books on such food-related topics as natural history, farming, food from different countries, cooking, gardening, and general science.

Use them in the book corner and also for display at particular times. The text is not of great importance for these purposes, but the pictures must be clear and attractive and illustrative of any points you're aiming to stress at the time.

Fruit and *The Egg* by Moonlight Publishing are two good examples of imaginatively produced natural science books suitable for young children.

Noisy Farm by Rod Campbell is also an imaginative 'first' farm book. Janet and Allen Ahlberg's *Funnybones* is a useful and popular book to bring out at certain times – see 'Bones, Dinosaurs and Fish', pages 75 and 80.

In case of difficulty, all the above-mentioned books, and other children's books, may be obtained from:

The Children's Bookshop
29 Fortis Green Road
London N10 3RT
Tel: 081-444 5500

They operate a 'Post-A-Book' service. Ring for details.

CHAPTER ELEVEN
Parties, Picnics and Outings

―――――――――

―――――――――――― PARTIES ――――――――――――

Parties mean crisps, sausages, cocktail savouries, paste sandwiches, jelly-and-custard, blancmange, ice cream, bright-coloured sweets, cakes with icing, orange squash . . . don't they? Well, they certainly used to. We would like to think that such a menu, especially if served to very young children, will soon be of only historical interest.

Amazing isn't it, that when we want to celebrate a happy occasion such as a child's birthday we seem to serve up *particularly* dubious fare!

We would be very angry indeed if a musician's visit to the nursery left some of the children deaf, or if a puppet show gave the children nightmares. How can anyone, then, justify giving the children food on any occasion that's detrimental to their health?

The quality of any nursery party food should be as high as at any other time. If individual parents wish to give their children high-sugar, high-salt, high-grease, low-fibre, low-nutrient, artificially-coloured, artificially fla-voured, mass-produced glop for their big birthday event, we can only regret it. We don't have to copy it on the grounds that the children may be used to it – or because we are.

More and more parents are trying, often against considerable odds, to prevent their young children from getting a taste for food that will undermine their health. We should applaud them and give them every scrap of support we can. We shouldn't be sabotaging them. Educational establishments like nurseries should be ahead, not trailing behind.

There will certainly be times when you want to put on a party in the nursery, but stick to your principles. Show the way.

So what will make it a party, then?

The same things that make any party a party! Namely, the atmosphere of excitement, the anticipation, wearing your 'best' clothes, the change in routine, the fun and funny hats, decorations around the room, decorations on the table and – plenty of absolutely delicious food and drink.

— But what can you do about a birthday cake? —

No problem. You make a toy cake, but with real candles, thus:

Fill a round toffee or cake tin with playdough. Cover the top with white paper and a double layer of white tissue paper, taped down all round. Put a cake frill round the tin and fasten with a pin. Buy five bright-coloured candles about six inches long and sharpen the base of each one to a tapering point with a penknife. Carefully cut holes in the tissue paper and push the candles firmly into the 'cake'.

Make 'candle roses' out of red or gold tinfoil paper, cut circles in the middle and drop over the candles. You have a cake! Bring it out on birthdays for the relevant child to light the correct number of candles using a long wax taper, while the other children – and any parents present – count, and then sing the usual song. They can all count again to see how many blows it takes to blow out all the flames – blowing *away from other children's faces* (lots of wax on these big candles).

In most situations, the cake ceremony (perhaps first thing in the morning with the mother or father present if that's possible), with maybe one special small item to eat later in the day, is quite enough for a nursery birthday. There is no need whatsoever for any nursery to feel it must put on any kind of 'birthday party tea'. Indeed, more time for play is a much better idea.

There's one problem you may have to deal with: in some nurseries, there's a tradition for the parent of the birthday child to bring in a fancy cake, and perhaps soft drinks and sweets as well. It is important when you are explaining to your parents that the nursery will be changing to a healthier style of eating, that you mention this matter. Once the cake has arrived it's a very tricky matter to refuse it. Be sure to mention what you *do* intend to do to celebrate birthdays. Remind the parents individually, well in advance, and invite them to their child's cake ceremony.

However, some parents do like to bring something for their children to eat with their friends at nursery, so suggest that if they particularly want to, then a little fresh fruit would be a good idea. When they see you are genuinely trying to do what is best for their children – and that the children like it – they may be more than happy to agree, and may welcome it as support for what they are trying to do at home. They might want to send half a dozen satsumas or rosy apples, or a small bunch of seedless grapes, a ripe guava, a pink melon, a box of strawberries, a slice of water melon, or a little pineapple . . . all real treats! The nursery can then be genuinely delighted to accept the parent's kind gift. (This is often considerably less expensive than the fancy cakes and such that the parents were bringing before.) If possible, involve the children in both the mathematical and fairness aspects of sharing the fruit.

Impromptu parties

These can sometimes be the most fun. Any occasion will do. For instance, if some children have been involved in a little boat or seaside project, then have a 'boat party' and eat the boats!

Quickly make the boats out of pieces of cucumber or carrot or courgette or celery, covered with curd cheese which could be used to glue on tiny sticks of carrot or celery for funnels. Children, staff and parents could all help to make the boats.

Sail them on a sea of clean blue paper or fabric. Have a shoal of fish swimming along: sardines on a blue plate – and seaweed: shredded lettuce here and there.

When it's ready, interested children can come to the 'party' and eat it all – boats, seaweed, fish, the lot! Sometimes fussy eaters are tempted to eat more when the food is presented in this kind of novelty way. Involve any songs or fun that you feel would be appropriate.

However, for times when you want to have more to eat than this, here are a few ideas. If you intend, at Christmas for example, to have a planned event that the parents will know about, plan your menu well in advance and post it up where everyone will see:

- to show that party fare *can* be nutritious too
- to give ideas – in fact a whole menu – for any interested parent to copy at home
- to demonstrate to parents who come to the party that the children will eat and enjoy healthy food.

The important thing with special occasion food is that it should look special. Get ideas for presentation from any conventional party book or from magazines. Copy their visual tricks and keep to your own ingredients!

FINGER FOODS

Savoury finger food	**Spreads and dips for the finger food**
strips of pitta bread	Iranian hummus (page 142)
fingers of toast	Israeli lentils (page 142)
commercial bread sticks,	mayonnaise
cheese straws or sablés	commercial taramasalata without
sticks of:	pink dye
cheese	avocado dip
carrot	peanut butter
celery	fish paté (page 142)
pimentos (red, green,	tahini
orange, yellow)	aïoli (mayonnaise with garlic)
courgette	cooked carrot mashed and orange juice
cucumber	
white radish	
seeded tomato	
radishes	
cauliflower florets	
celeriac	

Double-decker sandwiches

Alternate brown and white bread in each sandwich. Cut into squares, rectangles and triangles.

Have either the same filling or two different fillings:

Try Curd cheese or fromage frais with sunflower seeds, with slices of avocado in lemon juice and tomato strips, or with a little tuna and tomato or cress.

Try Peanut butter or tahini and a few sesame seeds with a little good quality honey.

Try Shredded lettuce and tiny, thin carrot sticks with mashed sardines and lemon juice.

Try Cold mashed scrambled egg with lettuce and chopped chives or mustard-and-cress.

Try Chopped prawns and mayonnaise with shredded lettuce and finely sliced celery.

Try Good Cheddar cheese in thin slices with any salad items and sprouted sunflower seeds.

Try Curd or cottage cheese, or fromage frais and lemon with lots of *very* thin slices of cucumber (why is it that lots of thin slices taste so different to two or three thick ones?); or with tomato slices; or with mashed avocado, tomato strips and sprouted alfalfa.

No need to butter the bread first when the fillings are tasty and moist.

Open-faced sandwiches

Make on bread or toast shapes, cheese scones, baps, crispbreads, matzos or crackers – great fun if you make them into faces.

Use Raisins, tomato strips and slices of vegetables for features.

Use Peanut butter, fromage frais, curd cheese or a good sunflower margarine as glue.

One-bite open sandwiches

Make on small circles of bread or small round crackers or cheese biscuits.

Use Curd cheese or fromage frais as glue.

Then put on One slice of tomato, or one slice of cucumber, a posy of mustard-and-cress, a few raisins in a pattern, a tuft of orange-juice-soaked grated carrot and a raisin, a bit of sardine or pilchard with a drop of lemon juice, a swirl of taramasalata, diamonds of red pepper etc.

Sweet dishes

Jellies and trifles, lollipops and ice cream can be excellent, valid, wholesome food, but you'll have to make them from scratch yourself. They are also hard work to serve fairly and clear away afterwards.

However, if you want to have a go for some very special occasion *and* you have plenty of willing helpers, there are some delicious recipes of healthy versions on pages 149–152. Lollipops can be made by freezing yogurt with fruit juice in plastic cups with a spatula in each one, and of course it would be lovely to offer the children treats like jelly and ice cream, knowing it would be doing them no harm at all!

However, you can serve much simpler things that a few adults can put together in minutes:

- Dried apple rings, pieces of dried apricot or pear can be got ready in advance and left, decorated with raisins, until needed.
- Middle- and Far-Eastern restaurants often put a platter of beautifully arranged orange, melon and (lemony) apple slices on the table at the

end of the meal. Copy this festive-looking idea; cover the plate with cling film and store in the fridge until needed.

- Serve a fruit salad, Greek-style: satsuma segments, pineapple wedges, tiny bunchlets of grapes (use seedless), fruit slices as above, mango slices, bananas cut diagonally into quarters and tossed in lemon juice, all arranged informally on large plates.

  If you can manage just a few black grapes (pipped), the colour contrast adds a great deal to the display. Don't put out strawberries unless someone is prepared to stand on guard until every single strawberry-lover has had one – and just one.

- A single strawberry (or raspberry, blackberry or any other treat) on a cushion of curd cheese, fromage frais or smatana on a small square of bread, one for each child (with a few in reserve), is a good finishing off treat, and a plate full of these looks extraordinarily good.

All in all, aim for small pieces of food, easily picked up, easily eaten.

Drinks

Mix your own drinks and avoid all the sugar and additives of the commercial kinds.

- Diluted fresh fruit juice – orange, apple, grapefruit, pineapple or mixed juices.
- Dilute concentrated pear juice (buy a two-litre container to cut down the cost, and use up over a period of time) – add enough fresh lemon juice to make a lemonade-like flavour. Serve from a large bowl with a ladle: nursery punch!
- Nursery Gluwein – as above, but use hot water. Delicious! Serve as a winter treat in large bowls with lemon slices floating on top.
- Milk
- Water, always, as a choice.

— Oooooh! —

That's what you should hear when the children first see the table of party food, however simple the fare. Long strips of snipped and twisted crepe paper, coloured streamers, fancy drinking straws are attractive, conventional, partyish things that will set the scene. Bunches of balloons, blown up by adults and hung up near the table are good, too.
Make sure the food itself is colourful and that its colour matches or contrasts with that of the plate. Try to notice if you're about to put the orange slices onto a pink plate and quickly transfer them to a green or white one! No party girl or boy is too young to deserve the enticement of beautifully presented food.

Nor are they too young for garnish – it really can put the finishing touches to a good dish and transform a plain-looking one. All garnish must be edible, however, because somebody will no doubt try it! If in doubt – don't.

- In summer, decorate plates of food as well as the table itself with edible flowers or their petals – marigolds, nasturtiums, chives, roses (unsprayed) – but again be careful, not all flowers are suitable: lilies-of-the-valley are poisonous, for example. (See page 92.)
- In winter, sprays of scrubbed and shiny bay leaves or of rosemary (from the nursery garden?) add a festive touch.
- Put halved orange or lemon slices all round the edge of a salad bowl or plate, or twists of thin slices on top.
- Scatter onion rings, chopped fresh parsley, spring onion tops or chives, or mustard-and-cress over savoury food.
- Arrange food on a bed of shredded outside leaves of lettuce.
- Radish roses, spring onion tassels and carrot flowers are colourful and fun – if you have the time to make them.
- If you are having a party, perhaps a quickie, an impromptu one, as part of an activity, the theme of the activity will suggest table decorations or colours, such as the 'Boat Party' described on page 118. After a story about rabbits and perhaps a sudden interest in them, have a rabbit party: green or earth-brown paper or fabric for the vegetable patch – perhaps Mr McGregor's garden itself – and the children can bunny-hop to it to nibble on bits of carrot and lettuce, celery and cabbage sticks, or little tomatoes.

NB: This might be an occasion to serve coleslaw – but a word of warning: some cooks think that 'healthy eating' means 'coleslaw'. It doesn't. Most children dislike coleslaw, at least in the way it is usually served in institutions. The pieces of vegetable are often just too thick and coarse to make pleasant eating, and many children don't care for the dressing, which may be of questionable value anyway. Lots of heavy chewing and not much reward.

If you do serve coleslaw at any time:

- Have only super-fine slices of cabbage and carrot and no big chunks at all. Try mixing in raisins and thin slices of apple.
- Mix with a little lemon juice and oil. Put it in mayonnaise only if you know your children like it.

Parties to celebrate festivals

We've already talked about this in Chapter six, but to recap: do make sure you celebrate festivals from a range of different cultures. Consult with the children's carers about how particular festivals might be appropriately recognized in the nursery. You may finish up getting some rather nice party surprises yourself!

PICNICS

These will probably be rather small-scale affairs, a snack-to-keep-me-going whilst on a little outing.

- Take anything mentioned elsewhere in the book that's dry, unsquashable and easily carried, i.e. tomatoes are out, apples are in.
- Remember you'll have no plates or cutlery unless you lug them with you – both ways!
- Remember to take plain water to drink. Nothing will quench thirst better. You'll need either individual flasks with *tight* lids or large containers and plastic cups or beakers. Remember, disposable plates and beakers can sometimes be washed and re-used.
- Any sandwiches will have to be well wrapped to keep them together. Any wet fillings will gradually work through the bread, though lettuce leaves will keep a sandwich tasting moist without this problem. Rolls stand up to punishment better than slices of a loaf.
- Cut fresh fruits into pieces if large, perhaps toss in lemon juice and wrap in cling-film to keep firmly together to prevent browning.
- If you're going to ask your parents to send packed lunches for a particular expedition, do ask for individual flasks or plastic bottles of plain water with tight lids, and *nothing else* to drink. Ask for the lunch to be sent in bags that the children can easily carry themselves.
- Whoever provides the food, you'll need damp cloths to wipe dirty/sticky fingers and faces, plus a supply of absorbent paper towels.

OUTINGS

Food outings are relatively uncommon compared with the usual kind of visit to the local zoo or park. It may sound mundane, but a trip even to a local market stall may actually be fascinating to many children.

Have a look round your neighbourhood and see what opportunities there might be for a little outing with a group of children. Visit shops, especially fresh fish shops which, amazingly, do not have *any* fish with fingers, but *heads* and *eyes!* These are very educational to visit. Look for stalls and shops that have a large variety of food on display.

This is what one nursery told us about shopping with children for special items for their meals:

Part of the fun for all of us has been in the joint shopping with the children for certain items. The three places we shop together are the market, the Nunhead wholefood shop and the local fresh fish shop.

Not only have the children learnt and provided amusing quotes, I have also learnt from the children.

The first time I took some children to the market to buy sweet potatoes, I was confronted by several items that fitted the description. As no labels were on them I told the children that I would have to ask the stall keeper which the sweet potatoes were, to which a three-year-old scornfully said 'That's sweet potato, that's green bananas and that's plantain, silly'. Oh well, out of the mouths of babes!

The fresh fish shop was a totally different matter and it was here that I was on a little safer ground!

The children viewed the fresh fish with a mixture of horror and fascination.

Fresh prawns did not have pips in them; the pips were really eyes – and the live eels! How did you get them in your mouth when they were wriggling?

The fishmonger has been extremely helpful in our education. He lets us all watch while he fillets and skins our fish and advises on preparation of some of the lesser known fish.

Samples from the shop are fun and the children seemed to either love or hate the prawns that they tasted.

Look into the possibility of visiting:

A farm, especially at seed-sowing or harvest time, or perhaps a city farm
Street markets or stalls; or shops that display food on the pavement
Garden centres
Cultural centres
Allotments
Private or public gardens with a herb and/or vegetable area or with fruit
    trees, or with goats, hens or ducks
A horticultural college
A pick-your-own fruit farm
A working windmill
A stately home with a kitchen garden
A bakery
An orchard

You may have someone connected with the nursery who would enjoy showing a private kitchen garden or allotment to a small group of appreciative people.

Ask around. One school made a trip to a Sikh Temple and were offered 'tasters' of all manner of delicious dishes, all beautifully served. Very educational and an unexpected bonus.

So you never know. Ask the parents, ask in your library, ask anyone who lives in, works in or otherwise knows your vicinity. Find out what treasures you may have right on your doorstep!

Recipes

Food for children (or anyone) should be nutritious and delicious. We believe the following recipes fulfill both these requirements. All are straightforward and economical. Butter and margarine work equally well in these recipes, although we recommend a good polyunsaturated margarine. Where a recipe is particularly good with butter we have said so.

Puddings

— Greek Lentil Soup —

This is the No-Time-To-Make-Soup soup. Also easy, cheap, nutritious and delicious!

20 servings
very cheap

500 g (1 lb) red lentils
250 g (¹/₂ lb) onions
lots of water
a little olive or sunflower oil
pinch of black pepper

Throw the lentils into about 3 litres (5 pints) of fast boiling water. Bring back to the boil.
Cook rapidly, adding more water every few minutes as the lentils absorb it. Stir regularly to prevent sticking.
The soup can be any consistency you like, but it's best moderately thick.
Meanwhile, slice the onions very thinly and cook in a little oil, covered, to completely soft. Continue cooking and allow to brown well.
Serve a little of this caramelized onion on the top of each child's bowl.

— Soupe à la Bonne Femme —

This means 'Soup in the style of a good woman, who knows how to make a terrific world-class dish out of next to nothing'. Known to every French housewife, it is perhaps the best vegetable soup of all. Easy and cheap – children can do most of the work, too!

10-12 servings
very cheap

500 g (1 lb) potatoes
4 carrots
2–3 big leeks
teaspoon sugar
30–50 g (1-2 oz) butter (the buttery flavour is good here)
fresh parsley
150 ml (¹/₄ pint) creamy milk

Clean the leeks carefully by cutting in half length-ways and washing under the tap to remove all soil and grit. Scrub the potatoes and carrots.
Chop leeks, potatoes and carrots into small pieces. Put into a soup pot with about 1¹/₂ litres (2¹/₂ pints) of water.
Add the butter, sugar, salt and pepper. Bring to the boil, then simmer about half an hour. Either liquidize or mash well with a potato masher. At the last moment stir in the creamy milk, heated, and scatter finely chopped parsley over.
This soup makes a good combined activity for children.

— Marrow Bone Minestrone —

See 'Bones, Dinosaurs and Fish' on page 80.

12 servings
cheap

This recipe is a particularly delicious form of a popular soup, and suitable for a main course. You need to make the stock the day before, so arrange to have something that's very quick to prepare, such as the Dutch Salad on page 131, on the day before you want to serve minestrone.

You can make do with a beef stock cube, but this soup is exceptionally good when made with real stock. As suggested on page 80, procuring and cooking a large marrow bone can involve the children in an interesting activity. The children can chop all the vegetables too. Anyway, here is a very easy way to make bone stock. You need to save vegetable scraps such as outside leaves and stalks of cabbage and cauliflower, leftover salad items, celery leaves and leek tops, – to help give (free!) flavour to the stock. Start the stock the day before.

EASY MARROW BONE STOCK
Place the chopped up marrow bone (or any beef or veal bones will do) in your largest pan of cold water. Add a teaspoon of salt and a teaspoon of vinegar. Cover. Bring to the boil. Simmer for three hours.
Add cleaned, chopped vegetable scraps.

Add a chopped onion, a bay-leaf, a few peppercorns and a good pinch of dried herbs.

Boil gently 20 minutes. Strain into a large bowl.

Next day remove the layer of fat from the top and discard or give to the birds. Then proceed with the soup:

2 onions
2 carrots
2 stalks celery
half a small white cabbage
1 potato
*1–2 cloves garlic**
500 g (1 lb) fresh or tinned tomatoes
tube of tomato paste
1³/₄ litres (3 pints) of good bone stock
sage, thyme, oregano (or marjoram), basil
a little fresh parsley
80 g (3 oz) wholewheat spaghetti
500 g (1 lb) minced beef or shredded ham or cooked haricot beans
Have grated cheese to serve

Chop up all the vegetables into thin pieces. Cook them in the stock, with the tomatoes, the tomato puree and the sage, thyme, oregano and basil (or use mixed herbs).

Break the spaghetti into short pieces. Throw into a separate pan of boiling water. Cook for exactly 10 minutes. Strain. Save in a bowl of cold water until needed.

When the vegetables are just done, crumble in the minced beef and boil, stirring for a minute or two, add the beans or shredded ham, and stir in. Stir in the cooked pasta.

Serve with grated cheese and fresh parsley. If using as a main course dish, serve brown bread and butter as well – good for mopping up the last drops from the bowl!

> *Don't be alarmed by the use of garlic: when cooked, it becomes very mild, soft and mellow, and almost disappears.

— Bortsch —

A northern variation of the minestrone recipe above.

Make as for minestrone, but omit the pasta and cheese. Add beetroot and yogurt:-

Cook about 4 round-shaped beetroot (not the elongated kind because they are too pale in colour) in a little water and save the water.

When very soft, peel and shred finely. When the main soup recipe is done, add the beetroot and the deep red cooking water. Serve plain yogurt or smatana or fromage frais to be stirred in at the table – and boiled potatoes or bread and butter if using as a main course.

In fact almost any meat or vegetables may be added to Bortsch, which has multitudinous variations.

— Quick Bortsch —

1 kilo (2 lbs) raw beetroot, scrubbed, topped and tailed
1 large onion, sliced
1 kilo (2 lbs) tinned tomatoes mashed
pepper
dash of tomato ketchup

Just boil up round beetroots and sliced onion in saved vegetable cooking-water until the beetroot is soft. Peel and shred the beetroots and replace in the water. Reheat with the tomatoes, ketchup and pepper.

Let the children stir in plenty of yogurt or smatana or fromage frais at the table.

Quicker still: buy cooked beetroot, peel and shred them and put into a little water along with other ingredients.

— Story-Turnip Soup —

See page 14 for how you might introduce this 'Tale Of The Turnip' soup.

easy
cheap
8–12 servings
1 – 1¹/₂ kilo (2–3 lb) turnips (not big old ones)
120 g (4oz) butter-and-sunflower-margarine
1¹/₄ litres (2 pints) milk
mixed spice
white pepper
about 3 tablespoons of milk powder
toast triangles

MAIN COURSES

First boil some water in a large saucepan. Scrub and peel the turnips. Young ones will give a better flavour – larger ones can taste very strong.

Put them into plenty of boiling water and cover.

Turn off the heat and leave about five minutes. Strain, rinse well under the cold tap and drain.

Roll them about in a teacloth to dry somewhat. Put into a soup pan with most of the butter and stir for a minute over heat.

Add the milk, spice and pepper. Cover and cook to tender, about 15 minutes. Stir in the milk powder to thicken, then liquidize. Pour back into your soup pan and stir in the rest of the butter.

If the soup is too thin, stir in more powdered milk.

Pour into individual bowls with a piece of toast in each one.

— Beanburgers —

10 burgers
cheap

250 g (8 oz) lentils (dry weight)
900 ml (1 1/2 pints) boiling water
bay leaf
1 medium-sized onion
6 oz carrots
3 stalks celery
1 clove garlic
small red or green pepper
oil for frying
1/2 teaspoon cayenne pepper
1/2 teaspoon mustard
1 heaped tablespoon of rolled oats
2 tablespoons tomato ketchup or purée

Pick over and wash the lentils. Then throw them into fast boiling water with the bay leaf, bring back to the boil, and simmer until soft. Stir from time to time, especially towards the end of the cooking. You should have a soft mass that will just hold its shape.

Meanwhile chop the onion, celery, garlic and carrots and cook in oil, covered, for about 15 minutes, or until rather soft. Chop the red or green pepper, add it to the other vegetables and cook another 4–5 minutes. Turn out the heat.

Beat the oats, cayenne, mustard and tomato ketchup (or purée) into the cooked lentils. Add the cooked vegetables.

Shape into ten small burgers, and coat in wholemeal flour or powdered wholewheat cereal. Fry in oil 2–3 minutes a side or until golden brown.

Eat with oven chips (page 140) or mashed potatoes, and a little green salad.

Variation: sprinkle with grated cheese and bubble under the grill.

— Greek Lamb and Tomatoes — with Rice

16-20 servings

2 shoulders of lamb, boned
500 g (1 lb) ripe tomatoes, sliced
a few slices of onion and garlic

Check the meat for any splinters of bone. Remove visible fat. Cut the meat into thin slices.

Arrange the meat in a layer in a shallow baking dish with a well-fitting lid, or make a lid with cooking foil.

Poke onion and garlic slices in between the pieces of meat. Scatter tomato slices over the top. Cover tightly.

Cook for two hours at gas 2 1/2, 310 °F, 160 °C, or until the meat is completely soft.

Serve with the following luscious rice dish.

— Greek Cinnamon Rice —

8 servings

1 1/2 teacups brown short grain rice
3 teacups hot water
1 tablespoon currants
15 g (1/2 oz) or so of sunflower margarine
2 tablespoons olive oil
pinch of pepper
1 teaspoon cinnamon

Fry the onion to soft and golden in the oil. Add margarine and rice. Cook for one minute, stirring.

Add water, salt, cinnamon. Bring to the boil.

Boil steadily for about eight minutes, or until the water has been absorbed, and little holes appear in the rice.

Tip into a warmed, greased casserole dish. Cover. Cook at gas 4, 350 °F, 180 °C, for half an hour.

Meanwhile soak the currants in hot water to clean and plump up.

Drain, and stir into the rice at the end of the cooking time.

— Dutch Winter Salad —

The recipe is interesting for its different textures – each ingredient has a totally different one – which can be pointed out to the children. A surprisingly substantial main course, it has to be the quickest, easiest meal with the least washing up ever!

12 servings
cheap
quick

3 dessert apples
3 large oranges
2 small sticks of chicory
350 g (12 oz) Gouda cheese
1¹/₂ litres (2¹/₂ pints) plain yogurt
6 medium potatoes

Wash but don't peel the apples. Chop them up along with the oranges and Gouda into the yogurt.

Cut the chicory across into thin slices and add these. Bake the potatoes. Serve the salad and half a potato on the same plate – the fruit-flavoured yogurt melts into the hot potato and so no fat is needed at all. Alternatively, serve the yogurt separately, so the children can see better what they're getting!

● Chicory is available from autumn to spring time only. It has an unusual and bitter flavour. It makes a good foil for the sweet apples and oranges, but slice it thinly

and mix it in well – don't leave whole leaves of it in the salad.

● Remember not to serve fresh fruit or yoghurt for dessert after this dish! Try a brown-rice pudding (page 149) or Honey Banana Custard (page 149) or Polish Cheesecake (page 151).

— Golden Sesame Slices —

An invaluable and popular vegetarian dish.

16-18 servings
very cheap

550 g (1 lb 3 oz) carrots
200 g (7 oz) grated cheese
150 g (5 oz) rolled oats
25 g (1 oz) wholemeal flour
30–50 g (1–2 oz) sesame seeds
50 ml (2 fl oz) milk
60 g (2 oz) melted sunflower margarine
pinch of black pepper

In a large bowl, mix the oats, flour, salt, pepper, half the sesame seeds and the grated cheese. Scrub and grate the carrots and stir in.

Add the milk to the melted sunflower margarine and stir in.

Press into a greased, shallow tray, about 30 × 22cm (12 x 8 inches). Sprinkle with the remaining sesame seeds.

Bake at gas 5, 375 °F, 190 °C for 25 minutes. Cut into slices for serving.

Eat with potatoes and either a green salad or cooked green vegetables.

● Also good cold as a snack.

— The Giant's Special — Beanstalk Stew

Can be used as as combined activity for children

15 servings

260 g (9 oz) raw haricot beans
150 g (5 oz) onion
150 g (5 oz) carrot
150 g (5 oz) potato

200 g (7 oz) courgettes
100 g (4 oz) French beans
400 g (1 lb) peeled tomatoes, fresh or tinned
1¾ litres (3 pints) vegetable stock
50 g (2 oz) wholemeal spaghetti
3 tablespoons sunflower oil
2 cloves garlic, crushed
1 tablespoon fresh or dried basil
slices of toasted wholemeal bread
150 g (5 oz) grated Gouda cheese

Soak the haricot beans overnight in cold water.

Next day, discard the water, rinse the beans, and cook 1–1½ hours, depending on the age of the beans, in the stock. Keep the stock for use later.

Dice the onion and slice the scrubbed carrots and courgettes.

Toss these in the the sunflower oil until slightly browned. Meanwhile, scrub and dice the potatoes, and add these to the saute along with the crushed garlic, and toss for 2–3 minutes. Add the cooked haricot beans and their cooking liquor, and the tomatoes.

When the carrot and potato pieces are almost cooked, throw in the spaghetti broken up into short lengths. After five minutes throw in the French beans, cut into thirds.

Cook five more minutes only.

The children can help themselves to triangles of toast and stir in pinches of grated cheese.

DID YOU KNOW

If you forget to soak the beans overnight, you can still save the day!

Just throw them into really fast-boiling *plain* water, bring quickly back to the boil, then simmer for *half* of their cooking time, or at least for 20 minutes. Drain.

Put into fresh water or stock and finish cooking.

— Meatless Pasties —

12 pasties

PASTRY
350 g (12 oz) flour,
230 g (7–8 oz) fat,
12 teaspoons cold water

FILLING
100 g (4 oz) tinned haricot beans, drained
1 onion, chopped
4 tomatoes, skinned, chopped
50 g (2 oz) sliced mushrooms
1 clove garlic, crushed
fresh black pepper
1 medium-sized potato, scrubbed and grated
2 medium-sized carrots, scrubbed and grated
milk or beaten egg for glaze
pinch of sage, thyme and fresh parsley
sunflower oil for frying

First make up the pastry and chill.
In a wide, covered pan, stew the onion slowly for about ten minutes.
Add tomatoes, mushrooms, garlic, potato and carrot.
Cover and stew for about five more minutes, stirring occasionally. Season with pepper and herbs.
Allow the mixture to cool somewhat. Stir in the beans.
Roll out the pastry rather thinly and cut into rounds, using a saucer as a guide.
Put a rounded tablespoon of filling down the centre of each pastry circle, and brush beaten egg round the edge.
Lift the pastry up either side of the filling and press the edges together securely.
Make a small slit on the top to allow steam to escape.
Brush all over with beaten egg. Stand the pasties on a greased baking sheet.
Bake at gas 6–7, 385 °F, 190 °C, to golden brown – 15–20 minutes.
Variation: Individual pasties are rather time-consuming. You could save time by adapting the above recipe to make a 'Pasty Pie' in a wide, shallow baking dish.

A TIP ON PASTRY MAKING

The nicest pastry to eat, and the easiest to make, contains very little water. Water makes pastry tough. Therefore, use only one teaspoon of water to each ounce of flour. But do use a little more fat than is usually given.
Three parts flour to two parts fat (as in the pasty recipe) is good. Use either 'wheatmeal' flour or half-and-half wholemeal and white. Unfortunately, soft margarines tend to make pastry too soft to handle easily, so hard margarine or butter, perhaps mixed with a little lard, is suggested. This may seem surprising, but we're recommending this recipe because

- It's the most delicious, melt-in-the-mouth one we know.
- It's easy to make – easier to roll out without cracking.
- It's very pliable, so it can be – and, indeed, should be – rolled out much more thinly than usual.
- Mouthful by mouthful, therefore, a little *less* fat should be eaten than with a conventional recipe.

* *

BUT

* *

Any pastry recipe is rather fatty, so we say 'Eat pastry just occasionally. When you do, make it the very best way you can.'

— Timatar Murghi —

This Indian dish is a great favourite with children. It is an authentic Indian dish, which is aromatic rather than spicy.

16 servings
easy

5 tablespoons sunflower oil
3/4 teaspoon ground cumin
1/2 teaspoon ground cinnamon
2 bay leaves
1/4 teaspoon black pepper
5 cloves garlic, crushed – essential!
1 inch fresh ginger, peeled and chopped
   or 1/2 teaspoon powdered ginger
1 kilo (2 lb) tomatoes, peeled, chopped (or tinned, partly drained)
16 small chicken drumsticks – fresh, not frozen
1 1/2 teaspoons salt
1/4 – 1/2 teaspoons cayenne pepper to taste
1/2 teaspoon garam masala
2 onions, peeled, chopped

Heat a large pot over a medium flame. Put in the oil. When this is hot, put in the bay leaves, cumin, cinnamon and pepper. Stir once then put in onions, garlic and ginger. Stir this around until the onion picks up brown specks.
Put in the tomatoes, salt, cayenne pepper and the chicken drumsticks. Stir, and bring to the boil.
Cover tightly. Simmer very slowly, stirring occasionally, until the chicken is completely cooked.
Sprinkle in the garam masala, stir and cook for about five minutes to cook the spice and reduce the liquid.
Serve with plain boiled rice. Allow 30-50 g (1–1 1/2 oz) per child, dry weight.

— Mixed Vegetable Curry —

12 servings

4 medium sized potatoes
4 medium sized carrots
2 medium sized onions
1 small cauliflower, broken into florets

1 red or orange pepper
a little sunflower oil for frying
1 level tablespoon curry powder or mild curry
    paste
a pinch each of powdered tumeric, ginger, cumin
    and coriander
1 tablespoon wholemeal flour
pinch of cayenne pepper, to taste – this is hot
    stuff!
teacup fresh orange juice
600 ml (1 pint) plain yogurt
pinch salt and black pepper
500 g (1 lb) tinned white haricot beans or chick
    peas

Peel the onions, and slice. Cook slowly in
the oil until soft, in a large covered pot.
Add the spices after five minutes of
cooking and stir in.
Meanwhile, scrub and dice the carrots and
potatoes. Dice the cauliflower stalk.
Stir the flour into the cooking pot. Cook
one minute, then stir in the carrot, potato
and cauliflower.
Add the orange juice. Cover. Simmer until
the carrots and potatoes are tender. About
half way through, chop the red pepper
into diamond shapes and add.
Just before serving, stir in the yogurt and
remove from the heat. Or let the children
stir the yogurt into their own helpings.
Serve with plain boiled rice, or with Yellow
Rice with Green Spots! below.

— Yellow Rice With Green Spots —

Cook the rice in your usual way, but:

1   In the pan you intend to cook the rice
in, cook some finely chopped onion in a
little oil first.
2   Stir a little turmeric into the onion and
fry for a few seconds.
3   Add water, stir, and when boiling, add
the rice and cook as usual.
4   Cook a handful of peas in a small
saucepan. Drain. Stir them into the cooked
rice just before serving.

This dish is also good on its own as a snack.

— Chicken in Peanut Sauce —

10 servings
inexpensive
easy

10 chicken drumsticks (or pieces of other meat or
fish)
juice of half a lemon
2-3 crushed garlic cloves   } mixed together
pinch of thyme
2–3 tablespoons sunflower oil

Toss the chicken (or meat or fish) in the
flavourings to coat completely.
Cook in the warmed oil, turning, to lightly
brown.

PEANUT SAUCE
1 large onion, chopped
250 g (8oz) crunchy peanut butter
500 g (1 lb) tomatoes, tinned, or fresh and
    peeled
600 ml (1 pint) water
pinch of cayenne pepper

Mix together the onion, tomatoes, pepper,
peanut butter and a little of the water.
Stir this into the chicken pieces. Stir in the
rest of the water. Cover.
Cook for 30–40 minutes, slowly, or until
the chicken is completely tender. Stir
regularly. Add more water if the sauce gets
too thick and begins to stick. Serve with
rice.
This is a West African dish and very good.
The delicious peanut sauce is known in
many countries.

— Wholewheat Pizza —

This is a particularly good recipe, relished
by children and adults alike.

6-8 servings

150 g (5 oz) plain flour, half wholemeal, half
    white
60 ml (2 fl oz) sunflower oil
60 ml (2 fl oz) milk
15 g (1/2 oz) fresh yeast or 10 g (1/4 oz) dried
a little oil
tomato sauce (see below)
a greased baking sheet, about 25 × 35cm (10 ×
    14 inches)

TOPPING

1 ball Mozzarella cheese or 5 oz Gouda.
30–50 g (1–2 oz) grated Parmesan cheese, or
Parmesan-and-Gouda
Any combination of the following: a few sliced
mushrooms, chopped parsley, black stoned olives,
shredded ham, flaked pilchards tuna or sardines,
tomato slices etc.

First make the dough: Crumble the yeast into a small bowl and add the milk heated to tepid. Stir and leave to dissolve.
Add the oil and the flour.
With your hands, make a very soft, pliable dough, adding more milk (or water) if needed to keep the dough soft. Knead for 2–3 minutes in your hands.
Leave to rise to double its size in your small bowl, covered with a damp cloth or plastic bag. Keep in a warm place.
Meanwhile, make the tomato sauce:

— Universal Tomato — Sauce

2 tablespoons sunflower oil
1 onion, chopped
bay leaf
2 cloves garlic, crushed
1 kilo (2 lb) tinned tomatoes or fresh ones,
  peeled
3–4 teaspoons tomato paste
pinch of sugar, pinch black pepper
thyme, basil, sage or mixed herbs

Cook the onion with the bay leaf in the oil and a drop of water until soft and yellow.
Add everything else, mashing the tomatoes down well.
Bring to the boil, then simmer, stirring from time to time to a thickened sauce.
This is an excellent and very useful sauce: use it on cod or chicken with rice and spinach, in lasagna or canneloni, with meat or beans, or in almost any recipe that calls for tomato sauce.

Punch down the risen dough, roll out very thinly to fit your baking sheet and pinch up the edges all round. Spread the tomato sauce evenly all over the dough.
Roughly slice the cheese and distribute over the sauce.
Arrange your other chosen toppings on the pizza and dust with Parmesan.
Bake in a hot oven, gas 7, 425 °F, 220 °C just above the middle of the oven, for 10 minutes.
Cool a little before serving to set the cheese. Serve with a tossed green salad.

— Spaghetti Bolognese —

Liver is highly nutritious. Many children dislike it. But in this recipe it is disguised in an extremely good and authentic sauce. Use half-mince and half-liver the first few times, but see if you can work up to using all liver without anyone noticing!

6-8 servings
highly nutritious
easy

60 g (2 oz) each of minced beef and chicken or lambs liver
or 125 g (4 oz) liver
2 large onions, chopped
2 cloves garlic, crushed
4 tablespoons sunflower oil
1 level tablespoon wholewheat flour
125 g (4 oz) mushrooms, sliced
a squirt of tomato paste (or ketchup)
pinch of basil and thyme
tiny pinch of sugar
tiny pinch of black pepper
600–800 ml (1¼ pints) stock or water
Grated Gouda to serve

Fry the onion in the oil until soft and lightly browned and add the garlic about half way through.
Stir in the meat and stir for a minute or two. Stir in the flour and cook for a few moments.
Stir in the stock; add everything else and bring to the boil.
Simmer slowly, stirring occasionally, to a good, thickened sauce.

Add more water as necessary to prevent sticking. Serve on top of the pasta on each plate. Allow at least 30 g (1 oz) of wholewheat pasta per child. Cook it exactly 10 minutes from when the water comes back to the boil.
Have grated Gouda cheese to scatter on at the end.

— Creamy Cod with Mushrooms and Mornay Sauce —

Fresh cod is often cheaper than frozen. Whiting and coley are cheaper still but must be skinned.
15–20 servings
highly nutritious

2 fillets of cod, each about 18 inches long
500 g (1 lb) mushrooms or mushroom stalks
1¼ litres (2 pints) good cheese sauce (see below)
1 finely chopped onion
1 tablespoon flour
1 tablespoon milk
1 tablespoon oil
about 4 tablespoons water or milk
fresh chopped parsley

Wipe the mushrooms and chop finely. Mix with the onion.
Cook quickly, stirring, in the tablespoon of oil, until they are noticeably reduced in quantity.
Stir in the flour, then the milk and cook for one minute longer.
Oil a large baking dish, and put in one of the cod fillets, skin-side down, diagonally. Cover with the mushroom mixture and then with the other fillet, skin-side up. Add a *little* water to the dish.
Cover the tin with a lid or with cooking foil. Bake at gas 5, 375 °F, 190 °C for about half an hour or until the thickest part of the fish is done. Don't overcook it. Dish up the cod 'sandwich' and coat with the hot cheese sauce.
Scatter a little fresh parsley over if you have it – don't use dried, which tastes completely different. Garnish with lemon slices.
The cheese sauce and the mushrooms

sweeten the dry taste of white fish substantially and make it more acceptable. Serve with potatoes and either green beans or peas.

— Easy Cheese Sauce —

100 g (4 oz) sunflower margarine
100 g (4 oz) wholewheat flour
600 ml (1 pint) milk
75–100 g (3–4oz) grated cheese
pinch pepper

Whisk flour and milk together in a saucepan.
Add the margarine and whisk over a medium heat until you have a thickened sauce.
Stir over a low heat for a minute or two to cook the flour well.
Stir in the grated cheese. Optionally, add a pinch of cayenne or mustard plus a dash of Worcester sauce for a livelier sauce.

— Hungarian Fish Casserole —

Fresh cod can be cheaper than frozen. Whiting and coley are cheaper still, but must be skinned
15 servings
economical
An easy one-pot dish

1 kilo (2 lb) cod fillets, skinned
25 g (1 oz) sunflower margarine
2 tablespoons oil
1 medium onion, sliced
1 clove garlic, crushed
15 g (½ oz) cornflour
1 teaspoon paprika
1 tablespoon tomato puree
250 g (8 oz) tinned tomatoes, drained, except for about 3 tablespoons of their juice
bay-leaf
black pepper

Cut the fish into chunks. Check for any stray bones.

Heat the margarine and oil in a large saucepan. Add the garlic and onion and cook to soft but not coloured, over a low heat.

Dust in the paprika and cornflour. Stir for one minute.

Stir in the tomato juice until it bubbles. Lower the heat, stir in the remaining ingredients with pepper to taste. Cover. Simmer for about five minutes, until the fish is just done. Do not overcook.

— Hearty Red Bean Stew —

A delicious traditional Afro-Carribean dish

12 servings
easy

550 g (1 1/4 lb) cooked red kidney beans
6 chopped tomatoes (canned or fresh, peeled)
600 ml (1 pint) vegetable stock or water
1 large onion, chopped
2–3 cloves of garlic, crushed
2 bay leaves
1 tablespoon chopped parsley
pinch or two of thyme
1 teaspoon paprika
180 g (6oz) chopped white cabbage
half a green pepper, chopped
1 tablespoon soya sauce
50 g (2oz) creamed coconut cut into small pieces

Fry the onion and garlic in the oil until lightly browned, then add all the other ingredients except the coconut. Cook until the cabbage is about half done, stirring occasionally.

Add the creamed coconut and a little extra liquid if necessary, stir well and simmer another five minutes.

— Spanish Tuna —

A useful 'unfishy' fish recipe. Either use tinned tuna, or, if your fishmonger can supply you with some fresh (not frozen) tuna you may be able to do it more economically.

If preparing fresh tuna, ask the fishmonger to clean it, then get rid of the strong taste by soaking in water with a teaspoon of salt and of vinegar for about 15 minutes. Rinse well.

Tuna is an oily and very nutritious fish, often liked by habitual fish-haters.

16 servings

1 1/2 kilos (3 lbs) tuna, tinned or fresh, prepared as above
tomato sauce (see page 135)
a large red pepper
a little oil

First make the tomato sauce, but stop cooking it before it becomes thick.

Then drop pieces of tinned tuna into the sauce and stir gently until warmed through.

(Fresh tuna should be partly cooked first by grilling or frying, then cut up into smallish pieces and finished in the tomato sauce. Cook it on very low heat, tightly covered, for about 20 minutes. Stir occasionally.)

Meanwhile, slice the red pepper fairly thinly, toss over a high heat in a speck of oil, then stir into the tomato sauce to finish cooking.

— Jamaican Chicken Chow Mein —

Not to be confused with Chinese Chow Mein which is different. It can also be made with minced beef.

8 servings
very cheap
easy and quick

500 g (1 lb) home-cooked chicken meat in small pieces
stock saved from cooking the chicken
500 g (1 lb) spaghetti or egg noodles
1 small stalk of celery, diced
1 small onion, chopped
1 teacup mixed, chopped vegetables (use frozen)
1 cup fresh bean sprouts
1/2 teacup finely shredded white cabbage
little oil for frying
light soy sauce*

Saute the chopped celery, onion and cabbage in a little oil.

Stir in the chicken pieces to warm through. Add the stock saved from cooking the chicken.

Cook the spaghetti or noodles with the mixed vegetables. Drain and add to the chicken mixture. Stir in the soy sauce to taste and the bean sprouts.

*Light and dark both look the same, so do this test before you buy: Tip the bottle upside down for a second. Light soy will run back quickly when you turn it upright. Dark soy will leave a dark stain round the neck of the bottle. Light soy is more authentic and unthickened with burnt sugar.

— Chinese Vegetarian — Fried Rice

8 servings
can be very economical – vary it to suit your purse and the season

100 g (4 oz) long grain raw brown rice, ready cooked and cooled
100 g (4 oz) mushrooms, sliced thickly
1 onion, chopped finely
1 carrot, scrubbed and sliced very thinly
120 ml (4 fl oz) sunflower oil
1 tablespoon light soy sauce
100 g (4 oz) peas (use thawed frozen ones or fresh)
3 eggs, beaten with a pinch of salt

Optional extra vegetables, choose one or more
1 green pepper, diced
1 red pepper, diced
a few spring onions, cut into 1 inch lengths
1 small leek, cleaned well, cut into 1/4 inch pieces
small piece fresh ginger-root, chopped into tiny pieces
100 g (4 oz) tinned bamboo shoots, finely diced
100 g (4 oz) mange-tout peas, cut diagonally into two or three
6 Chinese cabbage leaves, shredded finely
2 pieces broccoli, peeled, cut into small pieces

Have all the ingredients prepared in advance and cook at the last moment. Chinese food is best not kept hot or reheated.

Heat half the oil in a wok or large pan. Cook the chopped onion and carrot (and leeks if using), stirring over high heat for two minutes.

Add the other vegetables except the mushrooms (and Chinese leaves, if using) and stir-fry for one minute.

Add the mushrooms (and leaves) and stir-fry for one minute. Stir in the soy sauce. Turn out the heat. In a large saucepan, quickly scramble the eggs in hot oil, and tip in the cold, cooked rice. Stir to make thoroughly hot, then mix with the cooked vegetables. Serve at once.

— Fried Rice With Chicken — or Lamb

To the above recipe add cooked chicken or lamb, cut into small pieces, along with the rice. You can, then, omit the eggs if you wish.

A few drops of sesame oil mixed with the other oil is a nicely authentic addition – but expensive.

— Irish Stew —

12 servings
easy
cheap

1 1/2 kilos (3 lb) stewing lamb or mutton
1 kilo (2 lb) potatoes, scrubbed, thickly sliced
500 g (1 lb) onions, sliced
500 g (1 lb) carrots, scrubbed, sliced
450 ml (3/4 pint) stock or vegetable water
pinch of fresh black pepper
2 teaspoons fresh chopped parsley
2 teaspoons chopped thyme

Trim fat from the meat (feed to the birds in winter). Check the meat for splinters of bone and wipe over.

Place the meat and the vegetables in layers in a large stewpan, scattering the herbs and pepper in between.

Cover with stock and bring to the boil. Lower the heat and simmer, tightly covered, for about two hours.

— Quiches —

8 servings

There are many variations on this theme. For a 23 cm (8 inch) diameter quiche tin, here is a good basic recipe.

160–180 g (5-6 oz) good shortcrust pastry (i.e. pastry made with 160–180 g (5-6 oz) of flour. See page 133.)
about 450 ml (³/₄ pint) whole milk
3 eggs
1 small onion, sliced
1 tablespoon oil for frying
30–50 g (1¹/₂ oz) grated cheese
pinch of fresh black pepper

Fry the onion in a covered pan in the oil very slowly to soft. Add a drop of water if it begins to stick.

Beat the eggs well in a bowl and add the milk.

Line a 23 cm (8 inch) pie or quiche tin with thinly rolled out pastry. Sprinkle a little cheese over the base along with the onion. Put in your chosen filling (see below) and pour on the milk mixture.

Bake on a pre-heated baking tray at gas 5, 375 °F 190 °C, for 30 minutes, or until risen, lightly browned and set.

SOME SUGGESTED FILLINGS

Cheese and Tomato
Chop up about four tomatoes and add a little extra cheese.

Green and Red Peppers
Use about half a pepper of each colour. Slice very thinly, cut into thirds, blanch very briefly in hot water. Save the water for stock, rinse the peppers under the cold tap to set their bright colour.
Dust the top with paprika.

Spinach and Tomato
Cook 250 g (8 oz) of spinach and drain thoroughly.
Put eight slices of tomato around the edge of the quiche, sitting them firmly on the spinach so they don't swim around when you pour the milk in!

Mushroom and Lemon
About 50 g (2 oz) of mushrooms, wiped, sliced thickly
knob of butter
pinch of fresh black pepper
juice of ¹/₂ lemon

Saute the mushrooms in the butter and pepper over a very high heat for just a few seconds, so they brown without losing any juices.

Add in the lemon juice and toss for another second or two. If the mushrooms squeak when pressed with a spoon, they are done! Never overcook or they'll lose their juice, flavour and resilience.

Tip into the pastry, and rinse out the frying pan with a little of the milk mixture.

*Lemon and black pepper accentuate the taste of mushrooms

— Carrot Quiche —

This is a different kind of quiche, as the pastry is filled up with cooked carrots and only about half the amount of milk and egg mixture will be required.

about 250 g (¹/₂ lb) carrots, scrubbed, very thinly sliced
fresh parsley
wheatgerm
25 g (1 oz) sunflower margarine
little chopped parsley

Stew the carrots slowly in a covered frying pan in the sunflower margarine and a little stock or water, until they are cooked but not mushy. Stir in the parsley.

Put into the pastry shell, pour in the milk mixture, and scatter wheat germ on the top.

— Winter Vegetable Quiche —

Again, this is different, and you will need only about half the usual quantity of milk and egg.

about 250 g (8 oz) mixed vegetables such as:
an onion, sliced
carrots, very thinly sliced
cabbage, very thinly sliced
broccoli, peeled, broken to bits
4–5 thinly sliced Brussels sprouts
knob of butter
squirt of lemon juice
2–3 oz mushrooms

MAIN COURSES

Stew all the vegetables (not the mushrooms) in the butter and a little stock or water until cooked but not mushy.
Put all into the pastry. Pour in the liquid. Top with a few *thin* mushroom slices and a dusting of paprika.

— How To Cook —
Appetising Fish

1   Remove every single bone – many people avoid fish purely because of fear of bones.
2   Cook S L O W L Y, and
3   Cook as little as possible – until only just done. If you can smell fish cooking, it's probably being ruined – cooked either too fast or too long, or both.
4   Sweeten the taste of white fish with cheese, mushrooms, parsley, peas, milk sauces, ratatouille. . .

— How To Cook —
Appetizing Meat

Children often find meat hard to chew, so do make sure all meat is both thoroughly cooked but still soft and moist. So either:

1   Cook small pieces slowly in a casserole or sauce until they can be cut with a spoon, or,
2   'Steam–roast' the meat by covering it completely with foil.

Adjust the oven temperature and cooking time so the meat cooks as slowly as possible for as long as possible, to make it soft and succulent and to ensure it is completely cooked right through.
Allow the meat to set for about 10 minutes before carving. See also page 50 on cooking meat safely.

— How to Cook —
Appetizing Vegetables

Many children prefer the taste of raw vegetables to cooked, so don't forget to serve them raw sometimes, in salads or as finger food. Try Brussels sprouts chopped up in a salad – they taste quite unrecognisably crunchy and nutty!
When you do cook vegetables;

1   Cook at the last moment and serve at once.
2   Stir-fry them in minimum fat and a drop of water.
3   Or, throw green vegetables into fast-boiling water or vegetable stock and cook very briefly – or steam them.
4   Start root vegetables in cold water or stock and keep covered – or steam them.

— Oven Chips —

Avoid the high fat content of conventional deep-fried chips by baking them instead. It's an idea stolen from ordinary roast potato recipes, but you cut the potatoes into chip-shapes and cook in much less fat. Amazingly perhaps, the appearance and flavour is much the same as ordinary chips. Don't forget to call them chips!
Just cut scrubbed but unpeeled potatoes into good-sized chips. Heat a *very* little oil in shallow trays.
Toss the potatoes quickly in the oil to barely coat.
Leave to bake 15–20 minutes in a hot oven, turning once.

— Welsh Punchnep —

A traditional recipe in which mixed root vegetables are cooked together, then mashed with a knob of butter. Equal quantities of potato and turnip are authentic, but you could use celeriac, carrot, parsnip or swede instead, or add green peas towards the end of the cooking time. Swedes–carrots–potatoes make a good combination. The mash does not have to be completely smooth!

24 servings
cheap
easy

1 kilo (2 lb) potatoes, scrubbed, cut up
1 kilo (2 lb) celeriac/turnip etc. peeled, cut up
75–100 g (3–4 oz) butter/sunflower margarine,
or mixture
pinch of black pepper

Boil the vegetables together, then mash.
Yogurt or milk may be added to soften the
mixture. Eat hot.

— How To Cook Brown Rice —

8–10 servings

2 teacups brown rice, washed, drained
4 teacups fast-boiling water
a heavy saucepan with a well-fitting lid

Throw the rice into the boiling water.
Bring back to the boil. Skim. Reduce the
heat to the lowest possible. Cover tightly.
Leave to cook undisturbed for
      25 minutes (short grain rice)
      30 minutes (long grain rice)
The rice should be perfectly cooked and all
the water absorbed. No need to rinse. The
grains should be separate, and rinsing
washes away nutrients.
(See page 130 for an oven method)

— Wholemeal Bread —

This is a particularly delicious wholemeal
recipe, very well-liked. But you can make
bread without any salt or sweetening.

TO MAKE A LARGE (2 LB) LOAF
500 g (1lb 1 oz) strong, plain flour, roughly ²/₃
*   wholemeal, ¹/₃ unbleached white*
30 g (1 oz) fresh yeast, or 15 g (¹/₂ oz) dried
*   yeast or 1 sachet of instant yeast*
1 teaspoon salt
2 teaspoons molasses, black treacle or honey
180 ml (6 fl oz) hot water
about 180–280 ml (6–9 fl oz) cold water
a well-greased, large (2 lb) loaf tin

Pour the hot water onto the molasses in a
jug. Stir to dissolve.
Pour in about 180 ml (6 fl oz) of cold water.
Stir in the yeast.
Cover the jug and put in a warm place to
bubble – about 15 minutes. Meanwhile mix
the flour(s) and salt in a mixing bowl.

Stir in the bubbling yeast mixture and mix
with the hands to a *very soft*, moist dough,
adding as much of the extra cold water as
needed.
Cover the bowl (a large plastic bag put over
it is ideal), and leave to rise to about double
its size in a warm place.
Punch down. Knead very briefly, then
push well down into your greased bread
tin. Level the top.
Enclose in a large plastic bag and let rise
again to slightly above the top of the tin.
Bake at once in a pre-heated oven.
Cook for 15 minutes at gas 8, 450 °F,
230 °C, then for a further 40 minutes at
gas 5, 375 °F, 190 °C.
Tip out, and bake for 5–10 minutes more,
upside down and not in the tin, to brown
the underneath well. Test by holding the
loaf upside down in one hand and tapping
the underneath: if the bread is done, you
should hear a distinct hollow, knocking
sound, and be able to feel the knocking in
the hand that is holding the loaf.
Underdone bread is very unpleasant to eat,
so if in doubt – cook a little longer.
Cool on a wire tray. Eat when completely
cold – new bread is very indigestible.

VARIATIONS
Vary the flavour of your bread by adding
such things as:
    cracked wheat or bulgar
    grated cheese and a pinch of mustard
    sprouted wheat grains
    dried fruit and a pinch of mixed spice
TO MAKE A SMALL (1 LB) LOAF
Use 350 g (³/₄ lb) flour
175–220 ml (6–8 fl) oz water
15 g (¹/₂ oz) fresh yeast
Bake at gas 7, 425 °F, 220 °C for 23
minutes in a small (1 lb) loaf tin.
FREE-FORM LOAVES
You don't have to use a bread tin. Just put
a mound, or mounds, of dough onto a
greased baking sheet and bake as above.
FOR ABOUT 10 ROLLS
Bake small balls of dough on a greased
baking sheet at gas 7, 425 °F, 220 °C, for
about 12–15 minutes.

SNACKS

— Fish Paté —

very easy
very quick

drained sardines
curd cheese, or curd cheese mixed with fromage frais
lemon juice

Mix in any proportions. A high proportion of sardines will make a stronger tasting, grey-looking paté. More cheese makes a creamy-looking one with a milder flavour. Add lemon juice to taste.

> ### TIP! HOT PITTA BREAD
>
> Freeze the pitta bread.
> When you are ready to use it, take it straight from the freezer, make thoroughly wet under the cold tap and put immediately under a heated grill.
> Warm the bread about a minute a side. It should steam, open up, and taste like freshly baked bread. Slit one side to fill, or tear into pieces to eat.

— Pitta Bread Snacks —

Either fill pitta pockets or serve pieces of pitta bread with any raw vegetable or salad items plus hummus or fish or liver paté, cold chicken, undyed taramasalata, tuna, pilchards, cheese etc.

— Persian Hummus —

500 g (1 lb) tinned and drained, or home-cooked, chick peas
juice 1–2 lemons
1/4 jar tahini
2–3 crushed garlic cloves
pinch cumin (optional)

Liquidise everything in a little water.

— Israeli Hummus with Lentils —

500 g (1 lb) red lentils, cooked
120 g (4 oz) brown rice, cooked
1 large onion, chopped
2 cloves garlic, crushed
little sunflower margarine and oil
1 teaspoon curry powder
pinch of cumin, sugar and black pepper

Slowly cook the onion in the fat and a drop of water, covered, and after about five minutes add the garlic.
When the onion is quite soft stir in the spices and sugar.
Cook, stirring, for one minute, then stir in the lentils and rice.

— Milk-shake 1 (Lassi) —

A traditional drink to have with curry, or as a snack with a samosa, bhaji or sandwich.
Blend plain yogurt smoothly with milk or water.
Add a minute amount of cumin and of either salt or sugar.

— Milk-shake 2 —

Liquidise two hard-boiled eggs in 125 ml (1/4 pint) of milk

add
1 teacup powdered milk
1 teacup yogurt
1 teacup of fresh orange juice
few drops real vanilla
pinch of nutmeg

Blend well, then whisk in *475 ml (3/4 pint) of milk*.
Highly nutritious – almost a meal!
Try also adding a banana or any other soft textured fruit.

S N A C K S

— Tatale —
(Ghanaian Plantain Pancakes)

8 servings

6 over-ripe plantains (i.e. black almost all over)
1/2 cup water
3 small onions, finely chopped
pinch of pepper
160 g (7 oz) ground rice or flour
oil for frying

Wash and peel the plantains.
Mix to a smooth paste along with the onions in the food processor.
Turn the mixture into a bowl and beat in the pepper, the ground rice or flour and a teaspoon or so of oil.
Mix in the water and let stand for about half an hour.
Fry teaspoonfuls in a shallow pan in about 1/2 cm of oil. Drain well.

— Kelewele —
(Ghanaian Plantain Chips)

8 servings
easy
cheap

2 ripe (yellow coloured) plantains
pinch pepper
oil for frying

Wash and peel the plantains and cut into fingers and rub with pepper. Heat oil until very hot.
Fry plantains until well browned.
Eat as a snack or a dessert.

— Koosie —
(Ghanaian Bean Cakes)

8 servings
cheap

500 g (1 lb) cow peas or black-eyed beans, soaked overnight
1 egg, beaten
tiny pinch of cayenne pepper

1 medium onion, very finely chopped
1/2 cup water
groundnut oil for deep frying

Drain the soaked beans or peas. Strain.
Pour boiling water over the beans and let them stand for 10 minutes.
Rub the beans in the hands to remove skins and eyes (or buy beans without skins if you can), or use as they are. Wash, drain and grind in a processor with the onion and a little water or stock.
Turn into a bowl and mix in the cayenne and egg. Beat well to aerate.
Deep fry teaspoonfuls for about eight minutes or until golden brown and crisp. Drain well.
Serve as a hot or cold snack or even as a dessert.

— Potato Snacks —

Potatoes are familiar and popular as well as being nutritious, so it's worth finding ideas based on them. Here are a few suggestions:

— Potatoes-in-their-Jackets —

After baking, halve them, mash each half a little with a fork, stirring some sunflower margarine. Then, either:

1 Make potato nests: hollow out a little. Tip in a small egg. Return to the oven. Bake a few more minutes to cook the egg.

Or

2 Fork in any mixture of the following:
grated cheese
fromage frais
yogurt and a chopped orange segment
sour cream or smatana
cold scrambled/hard-boiled egg with mayonnaise
shredded cooked chicken or ham
chopped chives or watercress and yogurt

Strew a little grated cheese or chopped parsley on top (or, perhaps, a little home-grown mustard-and-cress. . .)

— Little Potato Cakes —

These can be a delicious cold weather snack:
Mix cooked mashed potato with a very little flour and some grated cheese or flaked fish. Traditionally shaped into little round cakes and fried both sides, these cakes may also be baked on a greased baking sheet in the oven until hot. The mixture could also be cooked in one piece and cut into squares for serving:

— Fish Cakes —

Not 'fishy' tasting, and sometimes a good introduction for some children to fresh fish.
Beat 100–150 g (3–4 oz) of cooked whiting or coley into 500 g (1 lb) of mashed potato with a teaspoon or so of flour.
Beat in fresh chopped parsley and a pinch of black pepper.
Coat with dried breadcrumbs or wholewheat cereal crumbs mixed with flour and cook as above.

— Cheese and Potato Cakes —

Beat 100 g (3–4 oz) of grated cheese into 500 g (1 lb) of mashed potato. Beat in a little cayenne pepper and Worcestor sauce. Coat with wholemeal breadcrumbs or wholewheat cereal crumbs mixed with flour and cook as above.

— Bubble and Squeak —

Don't forget this old favourite, if only for the name!
Cook extra vegetables in advance, so that the final 'bubbling and squeaking' is a quick job.
Chop some cooked Brussels sprouts or cabbage into the mashed potato and cook as above.
Crisply grilled bacon is a delicious accompaniment.

— Colcannon —

Almost the same as the recipe above, except that in this traditional Irish recipe, a little onion is fried in the pan first, before adding mixed potatoes and cabbage.
Or, beat in some chopped leeks that have been simmered in milk.

— West Indian Sweet Potato Salad —

Cook a whole, well-scrubbed sweet potato until soft. Either bake it or boil it. Slice fairly thinly.
Toss in a little vinaigrette. Leave to cool.
Mix with a small amount of mayonnaise.

— Stir-fry Chickpeas —

Sprout the chickpeas in the usual way (see page 132).
Toss them in a spot of oil in a shallow pan over low heat for a minute or two.
Add a little vegetable cooking water to the pan, put on a well-fitting lid, and cook very slowly for 8–10 minutes.
Delicious as finger food, warm or cold, and also very good mixed with baked beans.

— Things on Toast —

Besides the ubiquitous baked bean (heat the beans with butter or margarine, or butter-and-oil so you don't need to butter the toast), try:

- Cheese on toast – *cold* cheese is very good – it's not essential to grill it!
- Garlic sunflower margarine – melt some sunflower margarine, stir in some crushed garlic and add a squeeze of lemon juice. Drizzle over the toast.
- Lemon sunflower margarine – add lemon juice to melted sunflower margarine pour over.
- Mashed sardines – heat gently with a little oil and lemon juice. Mix with shredded lettuce on the toast.

- Tahini and honey – use a smear of honey to lubricate the dry texture of tahini.
- Peanut butter – try to find one that is made only of peanuts.
- Herring roes – gently cook them in butter-and-oil for two minutes. Add lemon juice and fresh chopped parsley. Mash. Spread on toast and cover with shredded lettuce.
- Fish paté – see page 142.
- Cheese and tomato – bubble the cheese under the grill. Add a few *thin* slices of tomato. Bubble briefly again.
- Very thinly spread yeast extract.

- Scrambled egg, hot or cold. Or try frying a little onion in the pan first – wonderful!
- Tomatoes – Boil up tinned tomatoes without the juice. Mash. Add a tiny pinch of sugar and pepper. A pinch of cayenne improves the flavour considerably, too.

NB Refer back to page 78 for ideas for the humble sandwich,
and to page 119 for double-decker sandwich ideas.
Scandinavian (open) sandwiches are often preferred by children as they can see exactly what they are getting!

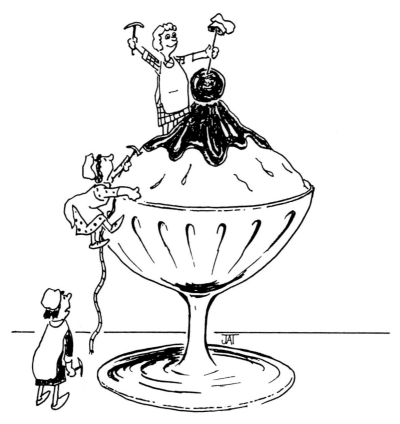

The Pudding Problem can be a difficult one to surmount.

Puddings tend to be made with refined white starches, sugar and fat, and thus present a challenge to cooks who wish to serve desserts which do not damage health. Recipes abound for so-called 'sugar-free' puddings, but they often contain such things as honey, molasses, muscavado sugar, 'raw' sugar, concentrated fruit juice mixtures and so on, which are not much better. So what should be done?

We suggest 10 strategies for dealing with the Pudding Problem:

1 Don't have a pudding! Horrors!! But if you serve a soup and a main course, the children won't need a third course.
2 Serve a delicious and filling main course, followed by a little piece of fresh fruit, or a small fresh fruit salad.
3 Add to the protein and calcium content of the meal by serving plain yogurt or fromage frais, and stirring in some chopped fresh fruit (see page 83 for ideas)
4 Collect recipes with very little sugar and very little fat.

5   Dried fruits and bananas are the sweetest fruits. Chop/mash these (in moderate quantities) into your low-sugar recipes and further reduce the sugar content.

6   Mix tart fruits with sweeter ones, for example,
     cherries with apricots
     figs with apples
     strawberries or raspberries with rhubarb
     chopped oranges with many things.

7   Use spices to cut the sharpness of tart fruit, for example,
     cinnamon and nutmeg with apples
     ginger with rhubarb
     mixed spice with apricots or brambles

8   If you must sweeten fruit, use ordinary fruit juice or dilute the concentrated kind. (Pear juice is useful as its flavour blends into that of the other ingredients.)

9   Change ordinary recipes to reduce their sugar-and-fat content, and to add more nutrients. (See page 151.)

10   Serve cheese and wholewheat crackers, or just cheese alone. Cheese and pears is a luscious and classic combination. Cheese has a cleansing effect on teeth.

— All-The-Year-Round — Fruit Salad

12–15 servings
cheap

2 big oranges
2 big dessert apples
2 grapefruit
2 bananas

Wash the apples, but don't peel. Chop everything up, the banana last, and toss. The grapefruit give a lovely tangy flavour. Prepare close to serving time if possible.

VARIATION
Top with Crunchy Dessert Topping (see page 151).

— Winter Fruit Salad —

12–15 servings
cheap
4 ripe pears
3 bananas
6 tangerines or clementines – or orange juice
(grating of nutmeg, optional)
Squeeze the juice and flesh from the tangerines. Chop the pears and bananas into the juice. Toss.
Utterly delicious, especially with smatana.

— Two Fruit Salad —

Combine any two fruits that complement each other, such as strawberries and oranges. (The oranges take on the flavour of the strawberries *and* make the strawberries taste better – as well as eking them out quite a bit.)
See page 83 for some other good fruit combinations.

— Fresh Fruit and Yogurt —

See page 83 for a list of ideas.

— Instant Banana Yogurt — Dessert

10 servings
cheap, quick, easy

3 bananas
1 large lemon
1 litre (1¹/2 pints) plain yogurt
3 teaspoons clear honey

Squeeze the lemon. Slice the banana into the lemon juice. Toss to coat well and put a little of this into each bowl.
Drizzle a very little honey over.
Add a spoonful of yogurt to almost cover the fruit.

VARIATIONS:

1 Sprinkle wheatgerm on the yogurt.
2 Sprinkle on a little Crunchy Dessert Topping (see page 151).
3 Use melon and ginger instead of banana and honey

— St Clement's Dried — Fruit Compote

A great improvement on the usual dried fruit salad. The orange juice makes it taste sweet.

6–8 servings
easy

250 g (8 oz) dried fruit salad mixture, or
  apricots and raisins
450 ml (³/4 pint) water, including a little fresh
  tea
pinch of cinnamon
1 orange
1 lemon.

Start this the day before.
Scrub the orange and lemon, then carefully cut off 2–3 strips of the 'zest' – the coloured part of the rind – and add it to the water along with the cinnamon. Use this for soaking and cooking your chosen dried fruit mixture.
Then, pour boiling water over the dried fruit and leave for 10 seconds. Drain. Serving is easier if you now cut the fruit into strips with scissors. Then put the fruit into the flavoured water and leave overnight.
Next day, bring to the boil and simmer about 40 minutes. Discard the peel.
Test. If the fruit isn't completely soft, cook a little more.
Squeeze the juice from the orange and add to the cooked fruit. Eat hot or cold with evaporated milk, smatana or yogurt.

— Fresh Fruit Compote —

Colour is the keyword here – it should not look like just another fruit salad. Avoid apples as they're too hard and pale.
Use at least one tin of strawberries and their juice to add colour to the compote.
Add a mixture of softish fruits in season or whatever you can find on sale very ripe and reduced in price. Look for bargain mango, passion fruit, cut melon, cherries, plums etc. Here is a basic, all-season version:

10 servings

500 g (1 lb) tin strawberries and juice
3 ripe pears
3 ripe bananas
2–3 oranges, depending on size
1 tin pineapple pieces in juice
a little fruit juice to moisten

Just slice all the fruit and put at once into the juice as you do it. Leave to macerate for an hour or more.

— Hot Fruit Compote —

As above – but heated just long enough to make hot. Don't cook it, or you'll just have stewed fruit.
Serve on its own or with Honey-Banana Custard (below).

— Honey Banana Custard —

Make up some custard in the usual way, omitting the sugar. Using two ripe bananas (i.e. with black-speckled skins) to every pint of milk, liquidize the custard and the bananas with a teaspoon of honey. Use as custard with any pudding.

— Honey-Banana Custard — Pudding

Chop slices of more banana into the custard to make a complete dish in itself.

— Greek Fruit Salad —

An arrangement of small pieces of fresh fruit on a plate. See page 121.

— Eastern Fruit Salad —

Similar to above. See page 120.

— Terrine Des Fruits —

12–16 servings

1200 ml (2 pints) tinned fruit juice (not fresh pineapple juice or the jelly won't set)
50–60 g (2 oz) powdered gelatine
a quantity of mixed fruits such as: 3 oranges, 3 seedless clementines, 3 bananas, 1 paw paw, 1 mango. Try soft fruit in summer time, kiwi fruit, ogan melons, etc. Avoid hard fruits like apple. Use whatever you can find that's a bargain at the time!

Sprinkle the gelatine evenly on 300 ml (½ pint) of the juice in a small saucepan. Leave to soften and change colour.
Very gently, and without stirring, heat the juice until all the gelatine has completely dissolved. Do not allow to boil.
Pour on the remaining liquid.
Pour into lightly oiled serving bowls. Leave to half set.
Prepare and chop your selection of fruit and pile into the jelly.

Leave to fully set in a cool place.
Either serve from the bowls, or, after dipping very briefly in hot water, turn out onto large plates – very spectacular!
Perhaps serve with Honey-Banana Custard (see left), evaporated milk or a little Yogurt Ice Cream (page 150).

— Brown Rice Pudding —

8 servings
cheap
easy

2 heaped tablespoons brown short-grain rice
600 ml (1 pint) hot milk
small can evaporated milk
2 heaped tablespoons sultanas or raisins
knob of sunflower margarine
a grating of fresh nutmeg

Wash the rice and fruit separately in boiling water. Drain.
Chop the fruit finely and mix with the rice in a pudding dish. Tip in all the other ingredients. Cook for three hours at gas 2, 300 °F, 160 °C, below the centre of the oven.
Break the skin and stir it in after half an hour, and once more half an hour later. Then let the skin form.

— Portuguese Rice Pudding —

8 servings

As above, but add:

the grated rind of two lemons
a pinch of cinnamon, instead of nutmeg.

When cooked, stir in the skin along with:

the juice of a lemon
another can of evaporated milk.

— Fruit Crumbles —

15 servings

CRUMBLE TOPPING:
Combine in a bowl:

PUDDINGS

500 g (1 lb) mixture of sunflower seeds, sesame
  seeds, wheat germ and chopped dried fruit
200 ml (12 fl oz) of fruit juice
2 tablespoons of sunflower oil

Put your chosen fruit filling evenly into a
baking dish and cover with the crumble
topping.
Bake at gas 4, 350 °F, 180 °C, until lightly
browned.

SPICED APPLE AND SULTANA FILLING
4 dessert apples
150 g (5 oz) sultanas or raisins, soaked in hot
  water for ½ an hour
50 g (2 oz) good margarine
pinch of cinnamon and fresh nutmeg

Wash and core the apples and cut into
rough but small pieces.
Stew them slowly with the soaked, drained,
sultanas in the sunflower margarine in a
covered pan until soft. Stir in the
cinnamon and nutmeg.

APPLE AND PINEAPPLE FILLING
As above, without the spices and with only
50 g (2 oz) of sultanas.
At the end of the cooking time, add a large
tin of pineapple pieces, or crushed
pineapple, in natural juice. (The juice can
be used to stew the apples in.)

APPLE AND BLACKBERRY FILLING
Stew the apples with 180 g (6 oz) of
blackberries and a pinch of mixed spice.
You may need to add a *little* sugar to this
one.
Experiment: try apricot and sultana with
mixed spice, raspberry and rhubarb with
ginger etc.
Serve with smatana, or yogurt or Honey-
Banana-Custard (page 149).

—— Ice-cream Pudding ——

A wartime recipe, very economical and
nutritious. The low sugar content has
further been cut by half. It makes a
delicious substitute for ice-cream and other
sweet desserts.
Serve it either:

- Chilled (not frozen) as an ice-cream
  substitute
or
- Warm or cold with a meringue on top as
  a special treat – and to use up the egg
  white

20 servings
very cheap

1200 ml (2 pints) milk
50 g (2 oz) sugar
120 g (4 oz) good margarine or butter
100 g (3½ oz) flour
2 eggs, separated
4 drops of real vanilla essence
few grains of salt

Cream fat and sugar to very soft. Beat in
the two egg yolks along with half the flour
and the salt. Beat well.
Heat the milk to fairly hot.
Carefully whisk in the milk and the
remaining flour bit by bit.
When smooth, return the mixture to the
saucepan, and cook very slowly, stirring all
the time, to a thickened custard. Bring
almost to the boil: it's done when when one
bubble breaks on the surface. Stir in the
vanilla.

—— Ice-Cream Pudding ——
with Meringue

As above, but make a meringue with the
two egg whites and a bare 50 g (2 oz) of
caster (or any) sugar. Pile in peaks over the
custard in a fireproof dish. Cook at gas ¼,
125 °F, 70 °C for an hour.

—— Yogurt Party ——
Ice-Cream

6–8 servings

60 g (2 oz) yellow sultanas
1 teaspoon clear honey
300 ml (½ pint) pear/apple juice
30 g (1 oz) dried apricots
450 ml (¾ pint) plain yogurt

Soak the fruit in the juice for 2–3 hours.
Roughly puree the fruit-and-juice in a
liquidizer.
Stir in everything else.
Freeze, stirring occasionally.
Soften in the fridge before serving.

Grandmother Rachel's Polish Cheesecake

An old Polish/Jewish recipe, easier to make
than most and still particularly delicious in
this reduced-fat-and-no-sugar version. An
excellent special occasion dish.

12–15 servings

250 g (8 oz) crushed digestive biscuits
90 g (3 oz) melted sunflower margarine
500 g (1 lb) curd cheese (don't use cottage
  cheese)
150 ml (5 fl oz) smatana, sour cream or yogurt
3 eggs, separated
75-100 g (3–4 oz) raisins/sultanas, plumped up
  in hot water
40 g (1 1/2 oz) sunflower margarine
few grains of salt
pinch of cinnamon
grated rind and juice of a well-scrubbed lemon
Large gratin dish or moule-à-manqué cake tin,
about 2 1/4 litres (4 pints) capacity.
Chop half the dried fruit roughly, leave
the rest and keep separate.
Line your dish with a thin crumb crust
made with the crushed biscuits and the
melted fat. Bake it for 3–4 minutes at gas 7,
375 °F, 190 °C.
Cream the 40 g (1 1/2 oz) sunflower
margarine with the chopped fruit.
Beat in the egg yolks, then the cheese.
Stir in the lemon juice and rind, the
remaining dried fruit, salt and cinnamon.
Beat smooth.
Whip the egg whites until stiff and
carefully fold in. Pour the mixture into the
crumb crust and bake at gas 7, 375 °F,
190 °C, for about 10 minutes.
Eat when completely cold.

Crunchy Dessert Topping

1 tablespoon clear honey
2 tablespoons sunflower oil
250 g (8 oz) rolled oats
50 g (2 oz) wheatgerm
50 g (2 oz) mixture of sunflower, sesame and
  pumpkin seeds

Gently melt the honey and oil together in a
small saucepan.
Mix with the dry ingredients. Spread on a
shallow baking tray.
Brown in a moderate oven, turning and
stirring occasionally until lightly toasted.
Cool.
Store when completely cold in an airtight
jar. Keeps well.

- Make a large amount and use it up over
  a period of time.
- This makes a delicious high-fibre
  breakfast cereal, too.
- The dry ingredients on their own make
  a good muesli.

Better Cakes and Puddings

Can't bear to part with a particular
favourite? Then:

- Change the flour to wholemeal.
- Cut the sugar content by 50% – it will
  taste the same! (But don't tell anyone –
  people taste what they *expect* to taste.)
- Depending on the recipe, cut the sugar
  further, or totally omit, and have
  liquidized or chopped raisins instead.
  (Unfortunately cutting the sugar more
  than just a little doesn't work with
  chocolate recipes or with carrot cake –
  unless you can add *lots* of dried fruit.
  Pity!)
- Use a good sunflower margarine in
  place of some or all of the butter. Use it
  melted in Christmas puddings and
  mincemeat instead of suet – and halve
  the amount.

VARIATIONS ON A BASIC CAKE RECIPE
Lemon cake: use grated rind and juice from a well-scrubbed lemon instead of water.
Orange cake: use grated rind and half the juice from a well-scrubbed orange, plus a squeeze of lemon.

Poppyseed cake: just mix a few seeds into the mixture with a little lemon juice and scatter a few on the top.
Fruit n' nut cake: add soaked raisins, sultanas, currants or chopped dates along with an ounce or so of ground almonds.

The Sling-in-the-Bin List

We recommend you get get rid of – and don't order – the following tooth-rotters, stomach fillers and artery-blockers:
- Commercially prepared desserts and cakes
- Commercially prepared burgers and pies
- Packet mixes, toppings etc.
- Tinned fruit in syrup
- Suet
- Synthetic fruit drinks
- Commercial fruit yogurts, jellies and ice-cream (make your own)

If you can bring youself to do it, try to sling out the following as well:
- Glacé cherries
- Golden syrup
- Cream, real or synthetic
- Condensed milk
- Biscuits
- Salted snacks

Budgeting

It is often stated that fresh fruit and salads and wholegrains are expensive. Yes, but nurseries that have changed to this healthier way of eating have found that the extra expense is balanced by *not* buying other types of food, particularly meat products. When large quantities of meat, ready-made desserts, orange squash, tinned fruit, custard and blancmange powder, lots of sugar and so on are no longer needed that saves money.

One nursery that made good arrangements with their local greengrocer, told us this:

> When changing our food policy, we telephoned the shop to explain. They were delighted to help and told us that by discussing what was in season, what the current prices were and what to plan within our menus during forthcoming weeks, we would eat better for less than expected. They have been proved right!

The added bonus is that we have a variety of food and vegetables: some we have never heard of or would never have purchased before.

This nursery found it beneficial, before changing over, to inspect closely every type of food normally bought and to re-evaluate it.

Another tip we were told was to buy unusual ingredients such as, for example, sweet potatoes or plantains, by doing a bit of forward planning with another local nursery and ordering the item together. This larger order made the local greengrocer happy to get them the food.

It all goes to show that with a little bit of determination, plus co-operation with all concerned, you can give children a fair deal in food.

Getting help

You can't do everything alone, of course. Even with a whole team of enthusiastic staff you will still want to get extra help and advice and information from outside sources. (See pages 114 and 115 for books on food-related topics for use with children.)

Who can you turn to?

Here are some suggestions:

Parents, grandparents and other carers Families have a lot of skills, often unrecognised or unappreciated. Encourage parents and other relatives and child-carers to get involved with your activities. Ask for help. See if they can give cooking demonstrations. Do they work in a shop you could visit? Do they grow food? Can they help with a festival? Start with something easy – say a taste-table (see page 55) which can be displayed and 'officially opened' at going-home time. Get them talking! Suggest a party or festival . . . Or maybe organize a talk. For that you may want a speaker, such as one of the following health professionals.

Health Education Officer or Health Promotion Officer These people work in the NHS to promote better health. They have resources like leaflets and posters, and they can help organize a talk for a group of parents or perhaps a training session for staff. Contact them through your District Hospital.

Community Dietitians These people work in the Dietetics Department of the District Hospital, and their role is to promote healthy eating in the community. They too may have leaflets and posters and can help to organize talks and training. They can give advice on making improvements to your menus and encouraging children to eat healthier diets. They can also help with advice on special eating needs.

Dental Health Education Officer or Community Dental Officer These people are also concerned with healthy eating, especially as it affects teeth. They can help with resources, talks and demonstrations on dental health. See if they can come and talk to the children as well as the grown-ups. Contact them through the District Hospital.

Environmental Health Officers These people work for the local Council and are concerned with, amongst other things, hygiene and food safety. They may have useful resources and information, and can give advice on kitchen practices and food storage (and wash basins and toilets, too). They can give advice about fridges and microwaves. They should be contacted if several children show signs of tummy bugs, e.g. vomiting or diarrhoea, or if you think you have been sold food that is unfit to eat.

Community Relations Councils (CRCs) Local CRCs can give advice and supply resources on various groups and activities in your area. Try also the Commission for Racial Equality (see Useful Addresses).

Religious and cultural centres If you are lucky enough to have some within visiting distance then it is well worth enquiring whether children would be welcome. See if the visit could be related to a festival. Some centres even make children welcome by offering home-made sweets!

Libraries Use them as much as you can, before they stop being free of charge! Librarians like a challenge and unused library services will be threatened with cuts or closure. So for their sakes and the children's, make libraries a regular part of the timetable.

Local shops, markets and restaurants Take the children out for trips. Perhaps bring the owners into the nursery, with samples of what they sell or do!

Primary Resource Co-ordinators Check your local Education Authority for materials and support they offer. Some have full-time officers just for under-fives and nursery support.

Companies, trade associations These, of course, must be treated with caution. Their motivation is to encourage consumption of their products and they may be blatant or (perhaps worse) very subtle about this. Sometimes it can just be a matter of cutting out a brand name from an attractive poster. But it can be much harder to counter half-lies like 'sweets won't cause any damage as long as you brush your teeth afterwards'.

Further Reading

*contains recipes

Science Activities from the 'Bright Ideas
For Early Years' series
by *Max de Boo*
Scholastic, 1990.

Sugar Off!*
by *Richard and Elizabeth Cook*
Pan Books Ltd., 1983.

Let's Eat Right To Keep Fit
by *Adelle Davis*
Unwin Paperbacks, 1979.

Let's Have Healthy Children
by *Adelle Davis*
Unwin Paperbacks, 1981.
Still the most readable and inspiring books
on nutrition for the layperson.

P.P.A's Cooking Round the World*
(booklet)
The Ealing Playgroups' Association 1986.

Creative Food Experiences for Children*
by *Goodwin and Pollen*
Center for Science in the Public Interest,
Washington DC, 1986.
Many practical ideas for schoolchildren of
all ages.

More Than Rice And Peas
by *Sara E. Hill*
The Food Commission, 1990.
A guide to food provision initiatives and
traditional eating patterns of ethnic
minority groups in Britain.

Nursery Cooking*
by *Molly Keane*
MacDonald & Co., 1986.
A delightful recipe book, illustrated with
exquisite watercolours by Linda Smith. Just
go easy on the puddings.

Living Without Sugar*
by *E. Lebricht*
Grafton Books, 1989.

**Children's Food – The Good, The Bad
and The Useless**
by *Tim Lobstein*
Unwin Paperbacks, 1988.
Takes a critical look at what parents and
children are being sold by the food
industry. Offers guidelines for healthy
eating and for getting things changed in
nurseries, schools and supermarkets.

**Feeding Time: How To Cope With Your
Child's Eating Problems**
by *Gillian Weaver*
Columbus Books, 1985.

Fun and Food for Playgroups* (booklet)
*West Midlands Pre-School Playgroups
Association*, 1987.

Useful Addresses

The Food Commission
102 Gloucester Place
London W1H 3DA
Tel: 071-935-9078

Action Against Allergy
24–26 High Street
Hampton Hill
Middlesex TW12 1PD (Please enclose SAE)

Asthma Research Council and Asthma Society
300 Upper Street
London N1 2XX
Tel: 071-226-2260

Hyperactive Children's Support Group
59 Meadowside
Angmering
Littlehampton
W. Sussex BN16 4BN

National Eczema Society
Tavistock House North
Tavistock Square
London WC1H 9SR
Tel: 071-388-4097

The British Dietetic Association
Daimler House
Paradise Circus Broadway
Birmingham B1 2BJ

British Diabetic Association
10 Queen Anne Street
London W1M OBD
Tel: 071-323-1531

The Coeliac Society
PO Box 220
High Wycombe
Bucks HP11 2HY

Pre-School Playgroups Association
11 Kings Cross Road
London WC1
Tel: 071-833-0991

National Society for Research into Allergy
PO Box 45
Hinckley
Leics. LE10 1JY
Tel: 0455-635212

La Leche League
B M Box 3424
London WC1N 3XX

Commission for Racial Equality
Elliot House, 10-12 Allington Street
London SW1E 5EH
Tel: 071-828 7022

STUDENT ASSIGNMENTS

Using the material in this book and the resources available in colleges and in nurseries and playgroups, students learning to be nursery staff, playgroup workers, nannies or child-minders should be able to undertake a range of different assignments relating to food. Here are some suggested projects:

——— CHAPTER 1 ———

1   What dangers to health are posed by the modern diet in Britain? In general terms, what changes do you think should be made to foodstuffs to make them healthier?
2   Write up an actual weekly menu of a nursery you know. In terms of health, how good do you consider this menu to be? Give reasons. Would you wish to change this menu? If so, in what way and why?
3   'A bit of what you fancy does you good'. Discuss this statement, with particular reference to children under five.
4   Find out who is responsible for planning the weekly menus at a nursery that you know. Then try to answer the following questions:

- What type of training in nutrition have the menu planners had?
- Was this training compulsory?
- How often is compulsory re-training on nutrition required for people who plan menus in your area, and what optional courses for professionals are available?
- What kind of training in nutrition are school cooks required have to have?
- How many people are usually involved in the planning of menus in a nursery you know?
- To what extent did the food actually served reflect what was written on the menu?

- Which people and/or institutions in your area are responsible for the nutritional guidelines of your menus?
- What conclusions do you reach about what you have discovered?

5   We know that babies should be breast fed for the first six months, but many are bottle fed nowadays. Try to find out why this happens. In particular, find out:

- Who in hospitals and in the community is responsible for the promotion of breast feeding? Who instructs and helps mothers to do this?
- All the different things that you think may influence a woman's decision whether or not to breast-feed.
- What part the manufacturers of baby milk formulas play in influencing mothers.
- If you can, talk to a mother who has breast fed her child about this experience. Ask her how easy it was for her to do this: who encouraged her, or discouraged her, who taught her, who (if anyone) explained the advantages of it to her?
- If it was your job to persuade someone to breastfeed her expected baby, what would you say?

or
- Suppose an expectant mother asked you whether you thought she should breast-feed her baby, what sort of answer would you give?

or
- Produce a sample pamphlet for expectant mothers on breast feeding, including title, headings, an indication of any useful illustrations and what you would consider to be a good text.

or
- Produce a video with others in your group that would be useful for encouraging and instructing expectant mothers in the art of breast-feeding.

CHAPTER 2

1   Imagine you have charge of a six-month old boy and a four-year-old girl in a private home. Both children were reared on commercial foods: milk formulas, tinned baby food and so on. The girl is used to a diet of fish fingers, sausages, chips and canned drinks. You have been given a free hand.

The parents are concerned about their daughter's diet, but tell you 'She won't eat anything else'.

Explain how you would deal with this situation. Give a few examples of the sort of meals you would give to each of the two children.

2   Find out how dinner time is organized in at least one nursery near you. Describe and comment on:

- The toileting and hand-washing organization.
- The attractiveness of the dining area.
- The way in which the food is served.
- The arrangements for staff dining.
- What happens to slow eaters.

Try to gather information from several nurseries and see if there is an overall pattern.

Note if any nursery seems to have solved any particular problem (e.g. children queuing up).

Draw diagrams if necessary to illustrate your points.

3   A friend tells you:

'I worked in a nursery once that went over to healthy eating and everybody hated it. Oh, they tried very hard – as from a certain day, they made sure that absolutely everything was beyond reproach, but the children just wouldn't eat it – well, it looked so awful – all those heaps of brown rice every day and horrible cabbage salads. We told them it was good for them, but they said they wanted some of the chips that the staff were having – oh goodness, the *staff* wouldn't eat health-foods!

Then the parents started complaining and demanded to know what was going on. It got very unpleasant. Do you know, the only time the children enjoyed their food was when we had a birthday and we had a cake and crisps! Well in the end they gave up of course. Had to.

- Make a list of all the mistakes this nursery seems to have made in changing their regime.
- How might these mistakes have been avoided?
- Describe how you would tackle the problem of a nursery which regularly served food of poor nutritional value, if you were in charge.
- If you were a new employee in such a nursery, what do you think you might be able to do to improve nutritional standards?

4   You have been asked to write a small leaflet to be given to parents just before their child starts nursery education explaining the nursery's policy on food. What information would you want to include?

Produce a sample leaflet, including title, headings, text and an indication of any illustrations you might want to include. *Or* produce a video on the subject.

5   What does the phrase 'poor animal husbandry' mean? Try to find out how *either* pigs *or* chickens are reared in Britain today. What effect do you think the conditions of rearing have upon

a the lives of the creatures themselves?
b the flavour of the meat?
c the safety of the meat for human consumption?

CHAPTER 3

1   You are working in a nursery that serves breakfast, mid-day lunch and then a tea for a few children who stay late. Plan one day's menus for this nursery. Then:

a Show how you would write this information up for the parents' notice board.

b Separately, list the dishes and explain why you chose each one.

2 Evaluate the following menu:

Breakfast	Rice Crispies or Cornflakes or Bran Flakes
	White sliced bread and strawberry jam
	Tea
Lunch	Beefburgers (bought, frozen)
	Oven chips (bought, frozen)
	Tinned spaghetti in tomato sauce
Tea	Jacket potatoes with grated cheese
	Bananas in chocolate sauce
	Milk

Item by item, say what you consider to be the faults and/or virtues of each one. Describe any changes you might wish to make. Write out your revised menu.

3 Someone tells you: 'A balanced diet should contain a bit of *everything*'. Discuss this remark with reference to:
a A two-month-old baby
b A nine-month-old baby
c A three-year-old child

4 Here is part of a conversation between a parent and child:

Child   I'm hungry!

Parent   It'll soon be dinner time.

Child   I can't wait. I'm *starving!* Can I have some chocolate?

Parent   No, you shouldn't eat between meals. Dinner'll be ready in an hour and chocolate will spoil your appetite.

Child (screaming)   It doesn't! I want some chocolate! I want some chocolate!

Comment on the replies of the parent. Re-write the scene with yourself playing the part of the parent. Write the rest of the

scene, including the ending. Perhaps make a video with others of your re-written scene. Make a list of items that you think would be suitable for a child's snack an hour or so before dinner.

5 Your nursery serves very good healthy food the children and staff enjoy eating. But three prospective parents are doubtful about the food that they have been told is being served.

Parent 1 says   I think you can go too far with all this health-food stuff. A lot of it is just a fad anyway. Children need *proper* food, not rabbit food. You need to have proper puddings too – fruit won't fill children up!

Parent 2 says   Sarah's got a good appetite, but she really only likes chips and fish fingers. I'm sure she won't like your sort of food. I know she won't eat the vegetarian food because we're not vegetarians.

Parent 3 says   This is good and I'm quite pleased, but it's not *completely* healthy, is it? I mean, to be really healthy you have to have just brown rice and muesli, don't you? And one of these puddings has some sugar in it – that should be honey.'

Explain in each case:

a The nutritional mistakes the parent is making.
b What you think could be said to each parent to allay their fears.

CHAPTER 4

1 Over a period of time try to notice how staff in a nursery in your area try to deal with children who are:

a 'Fussy' eaters
b Very small eaters

Describe how well the staff's strategies seem to work. Why do you think the children are 'fussy' or want to eat so little or are so slow?

2 Make a short study of a child who is unwilling to eat. Keep a record of occasions on which the child does eat more and what things seem to be putting the child off. Describe how you would deal with this particular child. Describe the apparent health and general liveliness of this child.

Keep a week's record of everything the child eats in the nursery. Try and discover the types and quantities of food the child has at home. Perhaps put this information on a computer.

3 Plan a day's menu for:

a A coeliac child
b A diabetic child
c A child with chewing and swallowing difficulties

State in each case the dietary principles you have used to construct the menu.

4 Try to find one or more adults who had a food problem when very young. Do some research: compile a collection of people's stories of childhood difficulties over food. In each case state:

- What might have started or perpetuated the problem?
- How was the problem solved?
- Did the problem continue into adult life in any form?
- Can you think of any way the problem might have been prevented?

——— CHAPTER 5 ———

1 Who is responsible for good food hygiene practices in nurseries? Why is food hygiene so important when one is caring for young children? What conditions favour the growth of food poisoning bacteria?
2 What dangers might there be using leftover food for another meal? Dinnertime has just finished and there are leftover jacket potatoes, tomato slices, lettuce leaves, cooked Brussels sprouts and some ham slices. Which, if any, of these foods might you keep for use the next day? Say how you might use them and what you might do (both today and tomorrow) to ensure maximum safety for each item. If you don't use an item, say why.

List some foods you would never re-use, and say why.
3 You are going to make some cheese scones with a small group of children. Explain in some detail how you would ensure high standards of food hygiene at each stage in the activity. To what extent would you involve the children in the hygiene aspect of cooking?
4 A mother of young children has asked you to cook a mid-day meal for the children tomorrow as she will be out. You have been asked to cook a frozen chicken, use part of a packet of frozen peas, re-heat today's gravy and yesterday's savoury rice. There are some potatoes in the vegetable rack as well. You've also been asked to make a fresh fruit salad but to include some tinned pineapple, leaving some pineapple for the next day; and to make enough custard for two days.

Write down how you would approach all of this from the point of view of food safety.
5 A friend tells you she has just started a lovely new job looking after a young baby, but she is appalled by the family's standard of hygiene in their scruffy kitchen. She said the family apologized for the kitchen but said it was going to be re-done in a few months' time. Your friend says she has counted ten things she considers to be health risks in the kitchen that should be put right immediately.

- Make a list of ten things your friend might have meant. Explain the hazards to health, especially to the baby, in each case.
- What do you think should be done about each of these problems?
- If it was your new job and you had found these problems, how would you deal with the situation, bearing in mind

that you don't want to lose the job, but are concerned about preparing food for the baby – and yourself – in such conditions?

CHAPTER 6

1   A nursery school teacher tells you 'We don't need to bother about multi-ethnic food here because we only have white children.'

- Discuss this statement.
- If you had a job at the nursery with this teacher, what do you think your approach should be?

2   What are some of the problems that might arise when a nursery is trying to introduce a good multicultural policy? Can you suggest some solutions? In what ways could food be:

a Part of the problem?
b Part of the solution?

3   a A friend tells you the nursery where she works always serves 'proper English food' and 'nothing foreign or exotic'. She goes on: 'Like today, our menu was:

Roast beef, potatoes and cauliflower
Rhubarb and apple pie and ice cream;
with tomato sandwiches and Scotch pancakes for tea.'

- Comment on your friend's statement.

b What should a nursery do if a parent says she doesn't want her child to be given any 'foreign stuff?' How might a nursery that wanted to introduce new foods start to do so?

4   You are working in a nursery in a city. The children are mostly Anglo-Irish but a quarter are Afro-Caribbean. There are also a few from Hindu families and a few from various European countries.

- Write the dinner menus for one week, bearing in mind

a The nutritional value of the foods
b The cultural backgrounds of the children

- What extra information about the children's background would it be useful to have when making the menus? How would you try to obtain the extra information?
- Try to obtain a weekly menu from a nursery with children from different cultures. What are the cultures? How does the menu reflect the ethnic mix in the nursery?

5   Choose three of the special celebrations below and imagine the nursery where you work has asked you to help plan an event to celebrate each of the three occasions.

Chinese New Year or Chinese Kite
    Festival
Shrove Tuesday
May Day
Jewish New Year
Divali
End of Ramadan (Id al Fitr)

In each case say, with particular reference to food:

- What sort of event would be appropriate to mark the occasion in a nursery ?
- What would be a good way of going about it?
- What you think would be the benefits of holding such an event?

CHAPTER 7

1   Make a list of art activities that nursery-age children could enjoy which involve food in some way. Try some of these ideas out and keep a record of:

- How well the activity worked and was enjoyed
- How you would improve it if you did it again
- Whether the activity provoked comments about the foods themselves

2   Set up a special interest table in a nursery which involves food, as a result of some incident, story or current interest. Try to get some contributions from the children for the table.

What activity or interest might lead from this table? Draw a diagram of the table indicating what was on it, or photograph it.

3   With some children make some toy food for *either* a nursery café or the home corner *or* some kind of food shop.

- Explain how you would introduce this activity.
- Explain how you would make sure the children know what the food they are going to make models of really looks like.
- Explain what arose during this activity that indicated possible follow-up activities.

——— CHAPTER 8 ———

1   You are to cook something with a small group of children. Write out the recipe, then say:

- Exactly how you will organize the session
- What you will do with the completed dish

Find an opportunity to carry out your plan. Write an evaluation of the activity.

2   What do you think are some of the benefits for children in cooking as (a) a combined activity, and (b) an individual activity?

- Say how you would organize a combined cookery session with a small group of children, with a particular recipe in mind.
- What safety measures would you take if the activity involved using knives sharp enough to cut up vegetables?
- Find an opportunity to carry out this activity.
- Write a short evaluation of the activity.

3   You have been asked to create a cookery resource area in the nursery. How would you begin to go about this? Then:

- Write a list of things you would want to put in the area.
- Say how these things would be displayed or stored.
- Draw a diagram to illustrate your use of the area.
- Describe the health and safety aspects of your arrangements.

4   a What would you say was the value of allowing children to cook individually?

- Write a recipe that would be suitable for six children at a time to make as individuals.
- Describe how you would organize this.
- If possible carry out this activity.
- Write down any changes you would make if you were to do the activity again.

b What would be the value to children of watching a short demonstration of some aspects of cooking?

- List the circumstances when you might want to do this.

5   Talk individually to:
a several children about what they liked or disliked about cooking at nursery school.
b adults who have been in charge of cooking activities in nurseries. Ask them, for example, about how they approached the activity from the health and safety, social, multicultural and nutritional aspects.

- What can you learn from these conversations?
- Give examples of how certain cooking activities can be linked to other projects and interests in the nursery.

——— CHAPTER 9 ———

1   What would you say is the value of encouraging children to grow things? What would you say to someone who was reluctant to grow things with children because she 'didn't know anything about gardening'?

2 You have been asked to create a 'green leafy area' inside your nursery, which should look attractive and also provide things to eat. You have a long, low windowsill, 18 inches deep, which gets plenty of sun, in the corner and next to a wall covered with pin-board. You can use two or three of the nursery's existing tallish plants for background if you want them. It is spring.

- Describe how you would go about the project.
- Draw a plan of how the windowsill will be laid out.
- If you can, try out your ideas in practice, keeping notes on what you do and how it turns out.
- Keep a record of activities you have observed involving children growing things indoors. Note the time of year the activity took place.

3 You want to brighten up a nursery's small asphalted play area. The area is bounded on two sides by school buildings with drain pipes and ground-level windowsills that get the afternoon sun; a third side is a high wall and the fourth is a low wire mesh fence with a gate in it connecting the nursery play area with the infants' playground.

- Describe what you could do to brighten up this area. A small amount of money is available but you know you will have to improvise quite a bit.
- Say when and how you would involve the children (and possibly parents) in setting up this area.
- As you might be the only person interested in maintaining the plants once established, how could you make the area as labour-saving as possible?
- Make notes on how local nurseries and schools have used their outside areas for plants.
- Investigate opportunities for putting at least one or two of your ideas into action.

4 As a result of a story, some of the children in your nursery are keen to 'grow something.' It is winter time. What things could they attempt? How would you organize it all? How would you use any food that was grown?

- Try out your ideas.
- Say how you would incorporate any of the ideas with other interests that are going on in the nursery.

5 Humpty Dumpty Egg Shells could be a suitable activity for Easter time or just to help the children enjoy the rhyme.

- List as many other occasions as you can when this activity might be suitably brought in.
- How could the things in the list below be used for nursery activities? Choose three and for each one list as many ideas as you can, with the idea of stimulating the child's interest in the item, learning something and having fun.

Beans or peas
Turnips or broccoli
Grains of wheat
A cabbage
Sandwiches
Milk
Nasturtiums or marigolds

Consider such ideas as language, music, gardening, artwork, cooking and eating in healthy and attractive ways, outings and mathematical development.

- Choose two of the ideas that seem to you to be particularly interesting and carry them out. Write a brief evaluation of your project.
- Perhaps combine your ideas with other people's to make a good-sized collection of ideas and make a poster to display them all.

——— CHAPTER 10 ———

1 In what way can cooking with children help their language development? Give an example of a particular cooking activity and say how it could encourage good language development.

2 Can growing things help children understand mathematical concepts? Give an example of:

a Growing something indoors
b Growing something outdoors

and say how each of these activities could encourage the children's mathematical development.

Say how you would go about these two activities.

3 Choose three short scientific experiments that you could do with young children. In each case explain:

a How and why you might introduce the activity
b What part the children would play in conducting the experiment
c In which ways the experiment would be useful for both language and mathematical development.

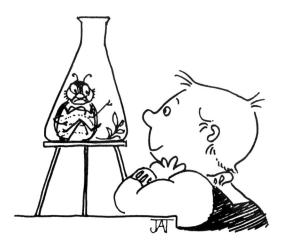

4 Make a list of up to six food activities that could be useful for teaching each of the following. Describe each activity briefly in note form.

- Fractions (halves and quarters)
- Counting
- Counting with ordinal numbers
- Ordering
- Shape
- Volume

Choose three of your suggested activities and say how you might attempt to bring out the particular mathematical point. How might you know whether or not the children grasped it?

5 How can food related-activities be integrated with music, dance and drama? Give some examples of how you might involve each of these three arts in three of the following:

- Making soup
- Shopping for ingredients
- Growing a runner bean
- Growing potatoes
- A fish activity
- Feeding the birds

Give some examples of how the activities you have suggested might arise.

——— CHAPTER 11 ———

1 You are helping to take a dozen four year olds on a little outing to a nearby city farm. You have been told there is a grassy area for picnics at the farm but no food or drink available there.

- How would you go about organizing a picnic lunch for this occasion? What planning would you do beforehand?
- Make up two different lunch menus for the occasion, each of good nutritional value and easily carried.
- Justify in detail the items you have chosen for one of the menus.
- Besides the lunch, what else would you take with you?
- What would you do with any leftover foods?

2 Pretend your group are food manufacturers trying to sell Crunchy Carrot Cookies. You want to give a party for children in a local nursery to persuade the children that carrots are wonderful. You have a small amount of money to promote carrots in general and your product in particular.

- The children will be offered carrots to eat and drink presented in a huge variety of unusual and tempting-looking ways. Make as long a list as you can of ways the carrots might be presented so they appeal to young children.

- Your firm will make up and adapt songs and rhymes, art activities and other fun activities for the party. Make a list of ideas in general, and go into detail on one of them.
- You have to think of possible table and wall decorations, models, dressing up, hand-outs and follow-up material for use by staff (you hope) later. Write out a list of the ideas.
- You need an advertising slogan about carrots in general that will appeal to young children. What will it be?
- Suggest ways in which the Crunchy Carrot Cookies might be

a Packaged
b Presented to the children

(TIP: Look at the methods food manufacturers already use to make their products appeal to children.)

Give three examples of how your ideas for promoting carrots could be extended by nursery staff to promote interest in healthy food in general.

3 Make a list of what you consider to be the nutritional faults in what is commonly thought of as children's party food. Why do you think many people serve such food? Why do many children eat it so willingly?

- Make up a menu for a birthday party in a private home for about eight 3–4 year olds.
- State the time of year of the birthday and how this affects your choice of menu items.
- Indicate how you would make the table look attractive.
- If you were expected to provide a birthday cake what do think would be a good idea?

4 Investigate how nurseries near you celebrate childrens' birthdays. Find out, for example, about:

- Any regular routine for celebrations
- Parental involvement
- The type of food offered: how salty, how sugary, whether home-made or commercially made
- How the pattern for the celebration became established
- How much the staff members enjoy it

Interview some of the children who have recently had a birthday about their views of the celebration.

Summarize your findings and draw some conclusions.

Index